Simply
NUTRITION

By Aimee Richmond B.S., M.D.

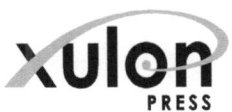

Copyright © 2016 by Aimee Richmond B.S., M.D.

Simply Nutrition
by Aimee Richmond B.S., M.D.

Printed in the United States of America.

ISBN 9781498492195

All rights reserved solely by the author. The author guarantees all contents are original and do not infringe upon the legal rights of any other person or work. No part of this book may be reproduced in any form without the permission of the author. The views expressed in this book are not necessarily those of the publisher.

Scripture quotations taken from the King James Version (KJV) – *public domain.*

www.xulonpress.com

Table of Contents

About The Author vii

Simply Nutrition, I 9
Simply Nutrition II, Vitamins 25
Simply Nutrition III, Minerals Calcium 49
Simply Nutrition IV, Foods 71

Bibliography 91

About The Author

As the daughter of a Presbyterian minister who had earned his PhD in Theology at Yale University (except for dissertation as he refused to write on the assigned topic "Emancipation of the Child" as he believed the Bible), Aimee Richmond grew up accustomed to learning, to the inquiring mind and to dedication to worthy endeavors. These attributes stood her well as she became one of the relatively few early women to study both nutrition-dietetics and medicine. In point of face, to this day most physicians do not receive training in nutrition.

Aimee earned the Bachelor of Science (B.S.) degree, majoring in dietetics-nutrition, in 1944, from Maryville College in Maryville, Tennessee. In 1948 she earned the Doctor of Medicine (M.D.) degree from the Woman's Medical College of Pennsylvania, which later became known as the Drexel University College of Medicine. Dr. Aimee actively practiced family medicine for a half century; she maintained her Board Certification in six states, finally "taking down her shingle" in 2003.

However, for this vibrant and continually dedicated physician, retiring from the active practice of medicine has not meant retiring from efforts to promote and assure good health. Her quest has taken two major and related directions. Both are centered on the effort to help people develop a better understanding of nutrition, its nature and sources and its relationship to wellness.

For several years, Dr. Aimee has affiliated with the nutritional products of Reliv International, a food science corporation headquartered in a suburb of St. Lois, MO. She has personally researched and used the products with emphasis on their consistent purity and effectiveness. Her results, along with thousands of others, give her great confidence that the food scientists at Reliv are contributing immensely to good health through the qualities of their nutritional supplements.

Her other quest has been to translate the mumbo jumbo of "scientific" language into ordinary terms which the interested person can comprehend; and which they can use to significantly increase understanding of food, nutrition, health and the interrelationship of the three. Thus she has written this little book, <u>Simply Nutrition</u>; sometimes it is called <u>Nutrition Made Simple</u>.

SIMPLY NUTRITION, I

*E*veryone eats or is fed. Foods have in them Proteins, Carbohydrates, Fats and Fiber. These also have vitamins and minerals. All have a place in keeping us healthy. When we eat at home or in a restaurant, we first choose the meat dish, then the side dishes such as vegetables including salads, starchy carbohydrates such as potatoes, rice, pastas such as spaghetti, macaroni, and noodles, and the fruit dishes and desserts such as pies, cakes, cookies, and ice cream or custards and whipped cream. Breads, biscuits, rolls, muffins, crackers, or corn tortilla chips are usually offered at restaurants and at dinners for groups. Butter is also available. Beverages are offered.

PROTEINS

Everything alive needs protein – people, birds, dogs and cats and all the animals in the zoo, the flowers, bushes, trees and grass in your yard, everything! We have lots of tiny things called cells which make up our bodies. Their walls have protein in them. Muscle cells are mostly protein. The heart is made of special muscle. The blood vessels, the arteries, veins and the itsy bitsy channels for blood called capillaries have another special kind of muscle cells. From the time we swallow food until the waste part comes out when we go to the bathroom, there are special muscle cells working for us. Our bones have a protein framework like a lattice or trellis similar to a screen in a screen door. The minerals calcium, phosphorous and magnesium attach themselves to this protein framework to make the bone strong and rigid. Protein is 3/4th of the dry weight of all cells of all matter.

The word protein comes from a Greek word meaning first. Protein has to be first in thinking about our food and about our bodies. Proteins are made up of a string of some twenty different amino acids, or organic compounds, which contain nitrogen as well as carbon, hydrogen and oxygen. Nine amino acids are called essential because our bodies can't make them and we need them to live. The 9 essential ones are histidine, isoleucine, leucine, lysine, methionine, phenylalanine, threonine, tryptophan, and valine.

Nine amino acids can be made in our bodies, so they are called non-essential. The 9 non-essential amino acids, which our bodies can make are arginine, alanine, aspartic acid, asparagine, glutamic acid, glutamine, glycine, praline, and serine. Two others, cysteine and tyrosine can be made by our bodies only if there is enough methionine and phenylalanine in our bodies to make them.

You can buy some of these amino acids and they can be helpful. As long as I take 500mg of lysine every morning I don't get fever blisters which used to give me a lot of trouble. Tryptophan has other uses and can be bought. I don't know anyone who has memorized all of the 20 amino acids that make up protein. Proteins which contain all of the essential amino acids are called "complete proteins"; these are most often found in meat, eggs, fish, soy, cheese (including cottage cheese), and milk.

However, it is handy to know that you can eat a protein which lacks certain essential amino acids and also eat another protein food which lacks other essential amino acids and the two together have the whole kit and caboodle. An example is matching whole grains such as corn, brown rice or whole wheat bread or crackers which are low in lysine and high in methionine with legumes such as beans, peas, and peanuts which are high in lysine and low in methionine. Together they make a complete protein. If you don't have a lot of money, corn bread and soup beans or brown rice and beans or peanut butter on whole wheat or whole rye bread or crackers can keep your body nourished with these important building blocks of protein.

Alcohol, more so in large quantities, can decrease the digestion, absorption, and use in the body of proteins. In the stomach there is a decrease in the digestive enzymes and acids. The pancreas has less ability to make the enzymes needed to digest proteins. The lining cells of the intestine are damaged by alcohol so absorption is decreased. The liver is less able to make proteins from amino acids due to alcohol.

CARBOHYDRATES

In 3000 BC in India sugar was made. Alexander the Great brought sugar cane from India to Europe about 327 BC. Hindus in India noticed the "honey urine" of the diabetic in the sixth century. In 1493 on his second voyage Christopher Columbus brought sugar cane to the New World. By boiling starch with dilute acid Kirchoff, a Russian chemist, changed starch to grape sugar (also called glucose or dextrose) in 1812. In 1844 Schmidt also showed that sugar was in the blood. In 1856 Claude Bernard, a physiologist, found glycogen (animal starch) in the liver of a well-fed animal. Carbohydrates are found in the form of monosaccharides, disaccharides, and polysaccharides. Mono means one, di means two, and poly means many. The sacchar part comes from the Latin word saccharum meaning sugar. Carbohydrates are made up of an equal number of carbon (carb) and water (hydrate) parts.

Although we can't live without protein, the biggest amount of our foods is mostly carbohydrates in the form of starch. We speak of the bread of life. Bread is a basic need world-wide. In some countries rice is the basis. When I was in Japan with a group of Americans, we were told that the word for breakfast was "morning rice" and supper was "evening rice." My Chinese friends liked to take a bowl of rice and place the Chinese food from the platter on top of the rice with chopsticks. I am very fond of brown rice and eat it a lot. In the United States, Canada and Europe the main grain is wheat. In the western part of South America mainly in the Andes Mountains region quinoa, a tiny grain, the seed of a weedy plant, is the staple grain; quinoa is the only grain which contains a complete protein. Corn is the main grain in Latin America. Tortillas are made with lime, which makes the nutrients in corn more available. Oats is one of the most nutritious grains, is great for breakfast, granola, and baked items. Barley is great in soups, but it can be made into cakes and breads. Whole rye is used in Germany and in Scandinavian countries as crisp breads and bread. Most rye bread in the United States contains a large portion of white processed wheat flour.

Potatoes are the main starchy vegetable in the US. Peru also uses and produces a lot of potatoes; they have white, yellow and red potatoes. Sweet potatoes contain a lot of starch and are very sweet and are delicious, almost like a dessert.

Highly refined grains and sugars were not part of our diet for 99.999 percent of human history. All vegetables and fruits are mainly carbohydrate. Eating lots of them keeps us healthy. An apple a day keeps the doctor away. This favorite saying also goes for all fruits and vegetables. The more colorful and tasty they are, the better they are for us. Isn't that nice? Beans, peas, lentils and peanuts which are ground nuts have both carbohydrate and protein. Tree nuts such as walnuts don't contain carbohydrate; they are protein and oil.

Avocadoes are tropical fruits which are about one third oil as well as carbohydrate. Honey and fruits contain sugar, also called fructose and levulose along with loads of vitamins and minerals. If someone doesn't want to eat his vegetables, but will eat fruit, not to worry. He can eat all fruit or all vegetable foods along with foods containing protein and fats or oils and get along fine.

Honey, pure maple syrup, molasses, sorghum syrup and stevia are natural sweets. They can be used instead of refined white sugar as sweeteners and will not rob the body of vitamins and minerals. When refined foods like white sugar, white rice, and white flour are eaten, they have to use minerals and vitamins to be burned in the body. Because they come in empty-handed they steal the vitamins and minerals they need from cells all over our bodies, and sooner or later the body complains by telling us it is tired and grumpy, can't think as well, and can't taste as well. I've seen people who have lost their taste of sweet so much that they use 3 or 4 packets of artificial sweetener in a cup of coffee. To me that would be ghastly sweet.

Glucose, fructose and galactose are monosaccharides. Glucose is also called dextrose, glucose needs insulin to be stored as glycogen in the muscles and the liver. Fructose does not need insulin to be changed into glycogen in muscles and the liver for future use for energy as glucose. Fructose does not cause as high a rise in blood sugar (plasma glucose) as glucose and sucrase, so can be used by diabetics to a limited amount (50-60 gm per day).

The disaccharides are sucrose, lactose, and maltose. Sucrose is usually made from sugar cane or from beets. Sucrose is the usual white sugar sold in stores and placed on tables and used in cakes, cookies, candies, pies and most sweets and added to many foods we buy including ketchup, soft drinks, sauces, sweet pickles and relishes.

Sucrose is made of glucose and fructose. Lactose (milk sugar), which is made of glucose and galactose is found in milk as its name suggests. Maltose is made of two glucose molecules and is formed form the breakdown of starch.

Cellulose and starch are polysaccharides. Human beings cannot digest cellulose. Cellulose is the thing that makes up the cell walls of plants. Our mothers would tell us to eat our roughage; this would be the parts of our food that is cellulose, not absorbed in the intestine, but acts like brooms to sweep the unused parts of food out of the body. Starch needs to be cooked so that heat and moisture can open up the plant cell walls and enzymes can reach the starch and the many glucose molecules can be released. When we chew our potato, oatmeal or bread, we also mix it with our saliva (spit). The enzyme from the saliva then starts digestion of the starch. In chemistry class, we spit in a test tube containing starch. Soon a test for glucose sugar became positive. In the intestine, juices from the pancreas mix with the food containing starch, and the enzymes from the pancreas digest the part of the starch to glucose to be absorbed in the intestine. Part of the starch is digested in the walls of the intestines into forms which can be absorbed. The disaccharides, sucrose, lactose, and maltose are digested in the intestine. The enzyme sucrose splits sucrose into glucose and fructose and splits maltose into 2 glucose molecules.

Lactase splits lactose into glucose and galactose. These simple monosaccharide sugars can be absorbed in the intestine. About half of the adults worldwide are lacking in lactase, and cannot tolerate a lot of milk unless it is fermented or changed into yogurt or kefir. They can usually tolerate about 3 1/3 oz. (100 ml) of milk without diarrhea or cramping.

Absorbed glucose is our main source of energy. As we burn it up we breathe out its products of carbon dioxide and water. After our energy needs are met, glucose can be stored in the liver and muscles as glycogen, also called animal starch. Most is in the liver. Insulin is needed for the glucose to be changed to glycogen in the liver and muscles. After the body fills up its stores of glycogen, the extra glucose is stored as fat. When glucose is stored as glycogen, 5% of the energy is lost and when glucose is stored as fat 28% of the energy is lost.

Between meals glycogen can be converted to glucose as needed. Glucagon and adrenalin are used to turn stored glycogen back into glucose. The brain and red blood cells use only glucose except when food is not eaten for a long period of time; then ketone bodies can be used.

When there is need for fight or flight, the adrenal glands make adrenalin and we get energy to escape danger or fight for our lives. Caffeine stimulates the adrenal glands to make adrenalin. Adrenalin stimulates the muscles of the skeleton to turn stored glycogen back into glucose. Glucagon causes the glycogen stored in the liver to turn back into glucose but has no effect on the glycogen in muscles.

Surgeon Captain T. L. Cleave studied Yemenite Jews and people in Iceland. He found that they had absolutely no diabetes or hardening of the arteries before refined sugar and refined flour were added to their diets. Twenty years after they were added these diseases were as common as in America. When Pima Indians, who have the highest rate of diabetes in the world, returned to their ancestral diet of seeds, nuts, berries, beans and lima beans, they were restored to health. Others who returned to their ancestral diets also returned to health. Refined sugar and refined grains exhaust the pancreas.

Associate Professor Somasundaram Addanki and his wife did not have diabetes while living in their native India. Professor Addanki, a biochemist and nutritionist at Ohio State University College of Medicine, began eating the typical western diet and became diabetic and suffered from diabetic impotency for six years. Then he stopped eating white sugar and white flour and was no longer diabetic. Larry Christensen, PhD did research at Texas A & M University that showed that some people were not sad or depressed anymore when they stopped eating sweets, candy and other foods containing white sugar and stopped drinking soda pop.

OILS AND FATS

Olive oil was one of the staples in many societies thousands of years ago. It is still valued today, especially in Greece, Italy, Jordan, Israel, and other countries. Olives are the fruit of a semitropical evergreen tree which can live a very long time. I have seen trees with very large trunks said to be thousands of years old. Olives are eaten in salads and with other foods. The oil is pressed out. I have seen ancient olive oil presses. Olive oil was considered so precious that it was listed as part of offerings brought to the temple. Olive oil can be used in cooking, in salads, and spread on bread instead of butter. It has also been used in skin softeners and in soaps. The olive branch was used as a peace offering.

Oils and fats are very important foods. They are very satisfying and keep us from getting hungry again quickly. We need them to survive.

Fats and oils do not dissolve in water. They can dissolve in ether and acetone. Some of the fatty acids in oils are needed by our bodies because our bodies are not able to make them; so we call them "essential". Essential fatty acids from oils are needed for all parts of our bodies to work. It is no wonder that eating nuts and fish is known to help people have good health and a long life because there are lots of these essential fatty acids in them. Not getting enough of these causes scaly skin, kidney, heart and liver problems, and poor healing of burns and wounds.

People gain excess weight because they are eating foods which signal the body to make insulin which then stores the extra food as fat. We do need some fat stores. Fat stores ae needed like a wallet to supply energy between meals. Fat is slowly digested and gives us more staying power to not get starved between meals. Refined grains such as white bread, crackers and pastas and sugar signal the body to make insulin which then deposits them as fat. Whole grains are digested more slowly and signal a much slower rise in insulin. Fats and oils and protein foods do not signal a rise in insulin, are more slowly digested and cause not appreciable rise in blood sugar. Eating enough of these and eating carbohydrates which do not signal a fast rise of insulin will go a long way in achieving a healthy weight for the person. By stop eating when no longer hungry and when one has had enough to eat is also helpful in having a healthy weight.

ALL THE "ESSENTIAL" FATTY ACIDS ARE IN OILS, NOT IN SOLID FATS.

Oils can get rancid by the effects of oxygen on them like the browning we see on a cut apple. We've learned to put lemon juice on cut fruit to prevent this browning. Vitamin C in the lemon juice is an antioxidant and does the job. So makers of foods to have a long store life got the idea of putting hydrogen into the oils which have some carbon atoms not saturated with hydrogen, and voila – solid fats which do not get rancid.

It is the oils which keep our hearts and blood vessels healthy, and it is too much of the solid fats which can cause the clogging of arteries in the heart and neck and legs. This can cause heart attacks, strokes, and legs getting tired on walking.

To explain how this works, let's look at what makes up oils. Oils are made up of fatty acids which are not saturated (full) of hydrogen. They may be mono-unsaturated or poly-unsaturated. Olive oil and canola oil are examples of mono-unsaturated fatty acids.

Fatty acids are carbon chains $CH_3(CH_2)nCOOH$; C stands for carbon, H stands for hydrogen, and O stands for oxygen. The COOH makes it an organic acid. The carbon atom has 4 bonds and can take both positive and negative atoms and bond to them. If a fatty acid is saturated, it has no double bonds between carbons; each carbon in the chain has 2 hydrogen atoms attached to it and its other 2 bonds go to the carbon atom on its right and on its left. The first carbon has 3 hydrogen atoms attached to it and its 4th bond goes to the next carbon atom in the chain. The last carbon atom has 1 bond to the preceding carbon atom, 2 bonds to an oxygen molecule, and 1 bond to the OH (hydroxyl) molecule. If a fatty acid is mono-unsaturated it has 1 double bond between 2 carbon atoms and only 1 instead of 2 hydrogen atoms attached to these 2 carbon atoms. If a fatty acid is poly-unsaturated it has 2 or more double bonds between carbon atoms.

POLYUNSATURATED FATTY ACIDS:

Both Omega 3 and Omega-6 fatty acids are "essential" and are polyunsaturated. Corn, safflower, sunflower and evening primrose oils contain omega-6 fatty acids. Salmon, mackerel, sardines, trout, and various sea foods contain one type of omega-3 fatty acids and flaxseed, soy and walnuts contain another type of omega-3 fatty acids.

Omega-3 fatty acids have the first double bond located at the third carbon from the end. Omega-6 fatty acids have the first double bond located at the sixth carbon from the end. Both Omega-3 and Omega-6 fatty acids are "essential" and are polyunsaturated. Corn, safflower, sunflower, and evening primrose oils contain omega-6 fatty acids. Salmon, mackerel, sardines, trout and various sea foods contain one type of omega-3 fatty acids and flaxseed, soy, and walnuts contain another type of omega-3 fatty acids. Omega-3 fatty acids have the first double bone located at the third carbon from the end. Omega-6 fatty acids have the first double bond located at the sixth carbon from the end.

When we eat fats and oils, they need to form into tiny droplets so that the enzymes can get to them similar to the fat in milk spreading through the milk. Bile from the liver helps in this process. Then they can be absorbed in the intestine (guts). Enzymes made by the tongue, the stomach, the pancreas, and the intestine work together in digestion of fats and oils. After being absorbed, fats and oils are transported to the liver. Some go by way of lymph vessels and others go by way of the portal vein.

SATURATED FATTY ACIDS ARE SOLID FAT.

In some Asian countries only 10% of their diets are fats or oils. In some European countries up to 45% of their diets are fats and oils. In the United States, it has been estimated that 30 to 40% of the diets are fats and oils. I would think that this would vary a lot among various ethnic groups and parts of the country. Some people believe that olive oil and the oil in nuts, avocado, and flax are better for our health. They need to be included in all diets including those of people desiring to lose weight.

FIBER

Another name for fiber is roughage. Our mothers told us to be sure to get our roughage. My grandpa had his health food; it was a combination of dried fruits including prunes. My dad told me about this. At camp we got a dish of stewed prunes every morning. No one got constipated.

After World War II Dr. Denis Burkitt and Dr. Hugh Trowell were working in Africa, and they noticed that certain diseases common in their native Britain were rare in people who lived in rural Africa. Dr. Burkitt asked missionaries to collect stools from Africans; he noticed the greater weight and the shorter time it took for the waste product to pass after food was eaten. These Africans had a large amount of undigested roughage, which we now call dietary fiber, in their food, totally 60 to 90 grams of fiber. This is similar to the Stone Age ancestors' intake of 100 grams of fiber per day. This use of high fiber foods is found among people living in the country in nations where they are making progress in politics, society, education, and developing industries and wealth mainly in their cities.

In rural Africa the diet has a large amount of whole grain cereals, legumes such as beans and peas, and root vegetables such as potatoes and yams. Heart attack, diabetes, and appendicitis were rare in Africans in the hospital in Uganda. In the Second World War in African troops who ate British army rations appendicitis appeared for the first time. At his 600 bed Uganda hospital, Dr. Burkitt noted that coronary heart disease was the cause of death in less than 1% (75% autopsy rate) of his patients who were African.

In 1976 Kehm, Anderson, and Ward showed that on high fiber diets, normal weight diabetics needed less insulin. Dr. James W. Anderson published a popular little book, Diabetes, a Practical New Guide to Heathy Living in 1981. In fact, non-diabetics used it as a guide. Following the high fiber, high carbohydrate diet 18 out of 20 normal weigh diabetics on less than 25 units of insulin were able to stay off of insulin for up to 4 years. In this diet 70% of calories were carbohydrate, 12% were fat, 18% were protein, and it contained 70 grams of fiber. On this diet, a 45 year old man dropped his cholesterol from 306 to 170 in 2 weeks and continued to keep it under 180 and a 53 year old man dropped his triglycerides over 2000 points from 3000 in 1 week, and in 4 months to less than 300, and he had a weight loss of 35 pounds.

In Dr. Anderson's diet, there is a great increase in whole grain bread and breakfast cereals such as oatmeal, brown rice, corn, barley, millet, rye, peas, lentils, root vegetables like potatoes, carrots, yams, sweet potatoes, parsnips, turnips, all fruits including dried fruits, and all vegetables including lettuce, cabbage and celery. Nuts are about half oil. Olive oil and canola oil are good choices. Cakes, pies, sweets and candies are greatly limited or avoided.

Fiber is the skeleton of the plant. Fiber makes the flowers, the trees and the vegetables able to stand up straight. The walls of cells are made up of fiber. People can't digest fiber so they don't get any calories from them. The cell walls are the carton or container holding the food. The fiber in the cell walls is mostly on the outside of the seeds, fruit, beans, wheat kernels, rice and other grains; it is often removed by peeling and in processing for grocery shelves. There are a number of kinds of fiber. Cellulose is found in vegetable fiber and wood fiber. Lignin is also found in vegetable fiber and wood fiber; lignin gets its name from the Latin name for wood, lignum. Pectin can be made from the peels of citrus fruits such as oranges, lemons, and limes. Pectin is used to make jams and jellies; it is also used medically to control diarrhea and along with plasma. Guar gum is used in making jellies used in pharmacies. Inulin is found in the roots of many plants and in tubers such as potatoes. Inulin is also used in a laboratory test checking how well the kidneys are working. It is also used in bread for diabetics. Inulin, cellulose, guar gum, and pectin are used to give bulk but no calories to food.

Some fibers are soluble, that is they can be dissolved in water; other fibers are insoluble and stay their separate selves and don't dissolve. Both are needed in our bodies. Some foods have both kinds. Oats and barley, though grains, have both kinds as well as vegetables and fruits. Whole grain breads and cereals, oats, whole wheat spaghetti and other pastas, brown rice, whole rye, and other whole grains are good sources of insoluble fiber.

Examples of soluble fiber include pectin, guar gum, mucilages, oat bran, barley, psyllium husk, legumes such as beans, peas, lentils, fruits and vegetables. Root vegetables such as potatoes, carrots, parsnips, turnips, and sweet potatoes are high in fiber, also nuts. Legumes such as beans and lentils are digested more slowly than cereal food or potato and more of them go into the colon (the large intestine).

Fiber helps the good bacteria grow in the colon. Bacteria are 80% water so the water content and the bulk of the stool (bowel movement) is increased. The good bacteria break down the fiber and make it more acid. When the stool is more acid, less cancer-causing substances (carcinogens) are formed. The increase in bulk also dilutes the substances that cause cancer, plus the stool passes out of the colon faster, so there is less contact with the lining of the colon. Guess what? Less cancer of the colon. People who live in the country in Africa have almost no bowel cancer. Seven Day Adventists have a higher fiber diet and have less bowel cancer.

Whole grains and other foods that haven't been refined slow down the rate that carbohydrates are absorbed. One way they do this is by the plant cell walls and bran layers acting as a wall making it take longer for the enzymes to get to the food. Gums and pectin slow down stomach emptying and slow absorption in the intestine. This results in a slower rise in blood sugar and in other substances.

An experiment was done to compare the form of food. This was done using raw apples with skins, apple sauce and apple juice. When raw apples were eaten, the rise in blood sugar was very gradual and didn't rise very high and then the fall in blood sugar was also very gradual and didn't cause any low dips in blood sugar. Apple juice caused a fast rise to a higher level of blood sugar followed by a rapid fall. The apple sauce blood sugar level was in between these two. The apples had all their fiber. The apple sauce had all the fiber but it was broken down and swallowed quickly. The apple juice had no fiber.

The people who ate the raw apples didn't get hungry again as fast as the people who drank the apple juice. Those who had apple sauce had hunger come again in between the two. There is less insulin response after eating apples than with the apple juice. The insulin response after eating apple sauce is in between these two.

Our ancestors ate 1 1/4 pounds of whole grain bread. Colas are 10% sugar by weight and contain no fiber, no vitamins, and no minerals, just empty calories. High fiber prevents overweight, heart attacks, diabetes, bowel cancer, appendicitis, and many other problems.

SIMPLY NUTRITION II, VITAMINS

Casimir Funk at the Lister Institute in London found thiamine (Vitamin B1) in 1911. He gave us the word vitamin. Casimir Funk was a poor and struggling biochemist who was studying pigeons. So, not having much money, he fed the pigeons hulls of rice scraped up off the laboratory floors. The pigeons didn't mind and were healthy and content. When he had a little extra money, he decided to treat his birds to the more esthetic and expensive polished rice. To his surprise the pigeons became lame. Convinced that their lameness was somehow related to their diet, he began investigating the difference between polished and unpolished rice. In the hulls of the rice he discovered a chemical compound known as an amino, which he later called the vital amine, later calling the substance vitamin. He cured his pigeons by feeding them a concentrate made from rice polishing.

Some vitamins dissolve in fat and are called fat-soluble. They are vitamins A, D, E, and K. They must be taken with food containing fats or oils to be absorbed in the intestine. The others, vitamin C and the B vitamins, are soluble in water and can be taken with or without food.

VITAMIN A

In ancient Egypt, the cure for night blindness was to squeeze the juice from cooked liver onto the eyes. This was noted in the Papyrus Ebers, the oldest papyrus still in existence. The ancient Greeks recommended eating liver as well as squeezing liver juice on the eyes.

We now know that the active ingredient in liver is vitamin A. As with other fat-soluble vitamins, vitamin A can be stored in the body in storage globules; 90% is in the liver, and the rest is in other organs. Storage of vitamin A is decreased when alcohol is taken over a long period of time even in relatively small amounts.

Food sources of Vitamin A include liver, other internal organs, eggs including the yoke, dairy, fish and liver oils of marine fish and marine mammals, e.g. cod liver oil. Food sources of beta carotene include carrots, dark green leafy vegetables, yams, spinach, tomatoes, yellow corn, and fruits such as papayas, ripe mangos and oranges.

Part of the vitamin A we swallow is in the form of retinol (vitamin A) and part in the form of beta carotene (provitamin A), which our bodies change into vitamin A for us. Vitamin A is absorbed into the blood stream and reaches the area where it is used faster than beta carotene. Vitamin E protects the Vitamin A from being destroyed by oxygen, both in the intestine before it is absorbed and in the storage globules in the liver and other parts of the body. Taking a good amount of both vitamins A and E helps all parts of our immune systems. Zinc is also needed for vitamin A to work.

Visual purple in the retina of the eyes is called rhodopsin; rhodopsin is made up of a protein and of a close relative of vitamin A. When light is shined in the eyes from headlights of an oncoming car, the vitamin A is used up and has to be replaced. If plenty is stored in the liver, this is almost right away. But if vitamin A isn't stored in the liver, we can't see in the dark and have a lot of trouble driving at night. Snow in the bright sunlight can do the same thing and we call this snow-blindness. Looking at computer screens, reading or typing on a lot of white papers can do the same thing.

Vitamin A is needed for cells to grow and for the manufacture of new cells. The cells that cover our bodies, such as the skin, and cells that line the inner surfaces of our bodies like the linings of the mouth, all of the digestive tract, the breathing passages, and the urinary tract must have vitamin A to work. If the breathing passages don't have vitamin A the cells can't make mucous and the little hair-like cilia which keep beating and cleaning out the breathing passages. These cells are lost and are replaced by hard scaly cells which can form cancers. Vitamin A is needed for taste, smell and hearing. A little girl in a small village was almost totally deaf when she was brought to a hospital in Israel. She was given good foods and vitamin A and vitamin E and after several months she could hear perfectly. Our bones and teeth need vitamin A. Without vitamin A children's teeth come in crooked. When a bone is broken, new bone cells grow to fill in the broken space and old bone cells are torn down. Without vitamin A new bone cells grow faster than the old ones can be torn down. Instead of a nice smooth healed bone, the broken bone is changed into a lop-sided shape. When we are under great stress, more vitamin A is needed to help the outer part of the adrenal glands make hormones to help us handle the stress.

Much of the changes of getting old are due to oxygen damage to our cells. Diets rich in vitamin A and beta carotene help promote long healthy lives by keeping oxygen from damaging cells all over our bodies, resulting in reduction of such issues as heart attacks, strokes, arthritis, and cancers. The pancreas has beta cells which make insulin; protecting these cells from oxygen damage prevents diabetes. An additional benefit: there is much fiber and water in fruits and vegetables which help to fill us up and we are not so likely to eat too much and gain too much weight. Food sources of vitamin A, such as egg yolk and milk containing some cream, also contain some fat which keeps us from getting hungry for a longer time and helps us stay at a healthy weight.

VITAMIN B COMPLEX

B complex vitamins work together so they need to be taken together. They do not have to be taken with food since they dissolve in water. Capsules containing B vitamins can even be swallowed with a glass of water. We have vitamin B1 (thiamine), B2 (riboflavin, B3 (niacin or niacinamide), B5 (pantothenic acid), B6 (pyridoxine), B12 (cyanocobalamin), PABA (para-amino benzoic acid), biotin and folic acid. Choline and inositol are vitamin-like compounds. All the B vitamins are found in brewer's yeast, liver, whole grain cereals and breads and pastas and brown rice. Good bacteria in our intestines can make some B vitamins.

B1 (THIAMINE)

Vitamin B1 works to change carbs (carbohydrates) into energy. The more carbs, the more B1 is needed. More is needed in exercise, in growing children, in pregnant women, and in women nursing babies. Also, more B vitamins are used up when people are going through hard stress and when sick with a fever. Having not enough B1 is bad for the heart, the blood vessels, the brain, the nerves, the muscles, the stomach and the intestines. The highest concentrations of B1 are in our muscles, also in our hearts, livers, kidneys, and brains. We can store B1 for only 9 to 18 days.

Whole grains such as oats, corn, barley, whole wheat bread, whole wheat spaghetti, whole rye crisp breads from Scandinavian countries and whole rye bread made in Germany, brown rice, and pork are good sources of B1. Smaller amounts are found in lots of foods. In cooking foods, B1 can be lost in the cooking water by high temperatures and by adding baking soda to the cooking water. It is OK to freeze foods as this does not destroy the B1.

In countries using rice as their main part of the diet, when rice began to be polished there was a huge outbreak of beriberi. This was around 1900 AD. Beriberi was first mentioned in the Chinese medical book, Neiching in 2697 B.C. Beriberi means "I cannot" in Singhalese. The person with beriberi is too sick to do anything, he 'cannot'. What foods are eaten, such as white rice, is the main cause for beriberi now in Asia.

If alcohol is served with the meal, less B1 is absorbed. Here in the U.S. and in Europe the main cause of a severe lack of B1 is alcoholism, an illness in which too much alcohol is the main source of the calories taken instead of foods containing vitamins. Although Wernicke's disease and Korsakoff's psychosis are mainly found in alcoholics, both can be found in people who have a severe lack of B1. If there is a less severe lack of B1, people have a lot of headaches, feel very tired, and out of sorts, cranky, and hot tempered.

B2 (RIBOFLAVIN)

Every cell in our bodies needs B2. Any time we eat any kind of food, whether carbs, protein or fats and oils, we need B2 to make them useful in the body. Vitamin B6 (pyridoxine) and vitamin B3 (niacin) need B2 to be present for them to do their work. A normal thyroid helps B2 to work. Riboflavin is yellow to orange-yellow; if we get more than we need, the extra shows up by making the urine yellow. If we don't get enough B2, we get sore tongues, cracked corners of the mouth, hair loss, fingernail and toenail problems, anemia, nerve problems, and stunted growth. Exercise does not increase our need of B2. It is not destroyed by heat. Women who are pregnant and who are nursing babies need more B2; breast milk has lots of B2. As with other B vitamins, B2 is needed to form new proteins from amino acids. It is absorbed in the intestines. We get a good supply of B2 when we eat egg yolks, milk, fresh meat, green vegetables, fish, cheese, wheat germ, liver, kidneys, mushrooms, avocados, beans, and whole grains.

B3 (NIACIN)

Niacin (B3) is needed for our cells to be made and to be repaired. It is needed for food to be turned into energy and for the brain and the nerves to work. B3 helps insulin work. Over 200 enzymes at work all over our bodies need B3. Heat, light, acid, and alkali do not destroy B3. The nicotinic acid form of B3 is used by the body to increase circulation in arms, and legs; also in hearts resulting in fewer heart attacks and deaths from heart disease.

Pellagra is a disease caused by a lack of niacin or tryptophan in the diet. In 1735 Dr. Casals in Spain diagnosed pellagra. It caused severe sickness in a population whose main diet had been corn for 200 years. Corn has very little niacin and tryptophan. But by grinding corn on limestone, the little niacin that is there becomes more easily absorbed in our bodies.

In the early 1900's pellagra became so widespread that it was an epidemic in the southeastern United States. Jails and hospitals for mentally ill persons were full of people suffering from pellagra. Here Dr. Joseph Goldberger, a bacteriologist, had the answer in 1922 when he discovered that the amino acid tryptophan could cure pellagra; and since tryptophan can be converted into niacin in the body he later discovered that niacin could cure pellagra. He had even presented his findings first in 1914, but there was tremendous opposition to his work. He died in 1929; by that time pellagra deaths had increased to 8 times as many as in 1914. Finally in 1939 the Council on Foods and Nutrition of the American Medical Association called for the fortification (adding) of niacin to white flour, white bread, and other staples. In the meantime thousands of people suffered and died of pellagra. A lack of niacin shows up in various problems. Being tired, lame-brained, down in the dumps, skin rashes in skin areas open to the sun, diarrhea, poor memory, being irritable, anxious, easily distracted, joints stiff and painful all can be from a lack of enough niacin.

The huge increase in the use of white sugar which contains no vitamins or minerals, only empty calories, but uses up B vitamins to be used in the body, has greatly increased the illness due to lack of niacin and other vitamins. So invite niacin to dinner. Liver is teaming with niacin and other B vitamins as well as other great nourishment. Meats, peanuts, other nuts and seeds, tuna, fish, poultry, eggs, milk, peas, beans, whole grains and brewer's yeast all have a good supply of niacin.

B5 (PANTOTHENIC ACID)

Our bodies use pantothenic acid, also called pantothenate by turning it into another substance, CoA (co-enzyme A). It is the anti-stress vitamin. CoA is vital to the health of the adrenal glands and to their making hormones needed to give you the emotional and physical energy to deal with any stress, from a bitter argument to a bitter winter, from a traffic jam to jam spilled on your shirt. Prisoners given a diet with no pantothenic acid become so exhausted and seriously ill that the test had to be stopped; they recovered slowly when given pantothenic acid. Children aged 7 to 12 in a refugee camp were so badly nourished that they were skin and bones and had bad teeth; their hair, eyelashes, and eyebrows had lost their color to snow white in many cases. On a good diet including eggs, vegetables, and fruit their hair color began to return in 3 weeks. Pantothenic acid has helped animals live longer, probably would help people, too. Studies have shown that it should be helpful in treating allergies.

Pantos is the Greek word for everywhere, and pantothenate lives up to its name and is found in almost all foods. It is brimming in whole, unprocessed foods. Whole grains like brown rice, oats and whole wheat, wheat germ, eggs, dark meat of turkey and chicken, liver, kidney, brewer's yeast, salmon and other fish, fresh vegetables, and royal jelly of bees supply pantothenic acid.

B5 can be partly lost in cooking and destroyed by acid and alkali. In freezing, vegetables lose 37 to 50% of B5. Canned vegetables lose 46 to 78% of B5. Processed and refined grains lose 37 to 74% of B5. Processed meats lose half to three quarters of B5. Unprocessed meats are better.

B6 (PYRIDOXINE)

B6 was discovered in 1944. It is needed in the use of amino acids and proteins in the body. The more protein eaten, the more B6 is needed. About 100 reactions using enzymes need B6. It is needed in the brain for signals to be sent over nerves, for example, serotonin. In both muscle and liver, B6 is needed to turn stored starch (glycogen) into glucose to be burned and produce energy. For B12 to be absorbed, B6 must be present. B6 is needed for us to have good immunity and for the hormones from the adrenal gland to work. B6 is needed to make several body chemicals. It helps zinc be absorbed. It is great in treating and preventing nausea of pregnancy.

If we don't have enough B6, the body makes too much oxalate, and this leads to kidney stones made of calcium oxalate. Lack of B6 can show up as sore mouth and tongue, cracked corners of the mouth, being out of sorts, down in the dumps, confused-not with it, anemia, nausea and vomiting, anger and convulsions. A severe lack of B6 can lead to anemia.

B6 is not affected by heat if in an acid environment such as tomato, but it is affected by heat if in an alkaline environment. It can be given by mouth or by a shot into a muscle. B6 is absorbed in the small intestine, and extra leaves the body in the urine. The liver supplies the active form of B6 to the circulation and other tissues. About 90% of B6 is in muscle.

Foods containing B6 include fish, turkey and chicken, meats, liver, brewer's yeast, soybeans, nuts, seeds, whole grains, wheat germ, bananas, plantains, figs, legumes, spinach, broccoli, cauliflower, beet greens, sweet potatoes, white potatoes, and asparagus. Alcohol increases the burning up of B6.

B12 (COBALAMIN)

Vitamin B12 is needed for the body to make red blood cells. In the lung red cells in the blood pick up oxygen which we breathe in, carry the oxygen in the arteries and capillaries to every part of our bodies. They then pick up the carbon dioxide waste product resulting from using the oxygen in burning glucose for energy, carry it back through the veins to the lungs so we can breathe it out. We see the oxygen loaded arteries as red and the carbon dioxide loaded veins as blue.

B12 by itself when eaten can do its work and be absorbed into our bodies only when there is available a substance made by the stomach, which scientists have named the "intrinsic factor" (intrinsic comes from a Latin word meaning inward). People who do not make this intrinsic factor or who have had part of their stomachs removed become anemic; then B12 can be injected into a muscle to do its job. B12 can be stored in the liver for 30 years, so signs of anemia may not show up right away after stomach surgery.

Before B12 was discovered, it was found that people with pernicious anemia due to lack of intrinsic factor could be helped by eating huge quantities of liver. In college in my dietetic classes we learned all kinds of recipes to get ground-up liver into tasty drinks and dishes; this was before 1944. In 1948 Beck and associates showed that B12 was the "extrinsic factor" (extrinsic comes from a Latin word meaning from without, outer) needed to make red blood cells. Also in 1948 2 groups of people separated out B12 from food (I would guess liver); these 2 groups were Rickes, Brink, and Koniuszy in the United States, and E.L. Smith and F. J. Parker in England.

B12 is also needed to make the protective sheaths (like our clothes) on nerve fibers. Because our bodies cannot make the myelin for these nerve sheaths (coverings) without B12, people get all sorts of nerve and brain problems when B12 is missing. Also B12 is needed to carry folate to where it is needed, and to store it. Folate is also needed along with B12 to make DNA, so changes in the body are widespread, not only in the bone marrow where blood cells are made, but in all lining cells of stomach and intestine and throughout the body wherever new cells are being made. Small amounts of B12 go into bile but are absorbed again in the small intestine. A tiny amount goes out in the urine. Lack of B12 may also show up in walking with feet far apart, unsteadiness in walking, being very tired, mental slowness, loss of memory, mixed up, down in the dumps and other nerve problems, as well as anemia with large pale red blood cells. The reason for the name pernicious (deadly, fatal) anemia is that people died of it.

Sources of B12 include liver, meats, eggs, dairy products, brewer's yeast, fish, kidneys, oysters, and shell-fish. It is absent in all plant foods. If the stomach is not making the substance needed for B12 to be absorbed, B12 may be given by injection. A nasal gel is available.

OTHER MEMBERS OF THE B COMPLEX

FOLIC ACID

Folic Acid (Folate) got its name because it was found in a leafy vegetable, spinach by Mitchell and coworkers in 1941. Folate is needed to allow cells to divide and make new cells including red blood cells and to make amino acids which go together to make proteins such as meat (muscles in people and animals). Our DNA and RNA in all our cells depend on folate.

A lack of folic acid in early pregnancy is the cause of Spina Bifida. I have had a patient who had Spina Bifida: this is there at birth; the spinal cord pushes out through an opening in the backbone where the arches of the backbone don't meet as they are supposed to. The person can't move his legs properly; sometimes he or she can't keep the urine from coming out and has to wear diapers. Now all vitamins given for pregnant ladies contain folic acid. I advised ladies wanting to have a baby to start taking these vitamins before they got pregnant, because the damage is done in very early pregnancy, sometimes before it is known that there is a pregnancy.

Folate is absorbed in the intestine. About half of the stored folate is in the liver and a small amount goes out in the bile. A tiny amount goes out in the urine because the kidneys absorb most of it back. When a large amount of alcohol is taken in, less food containing folate is eaten, less is absorbed, more is lost, more is destroyed, yet more is needed. Very many people in the U.S. don't get enough folate. If people don't get enough folate, they are pale, tired, dizzy, short of breath, can't concentrate, may not feel like eating, may even feel sick to the stomach and have running off of the bowels. Because folate is needed to make the DNA for new brain cells, they may not remember where they parked their cars. You can't get too much folate as the body gets rid of what it doesn't need.

How do you get folate? It is in liver, heart, kidney, yeast, fresh green vegetables and fruit, wheat germ, dried peas and beans, and grains which have had folate added to them. Eating one fresh fruit or vegetable daily can prevent the problems of folate deficiency (lack of folate).

BIOTIN

Biotin is a water soluble vitamin, part of the B complex: it is sometimes referred to as vitamin H (German H for Haut, skin). Biotin works in the process whereby fatty acids are used in making the stores of fat needed for long time fuel for the body. Energy may be stored as glycogen (animal starch) and biotin helps turn this into glucose to use as fuel, especially in the brain and in the red blood cells. Biotin is needed in using fatty acids, carbohydrates, protein, folic acid, pantothenic acid, and B12. It is needed for the health of skin, hair, nerves, bone marrow, sex glands, and for good body immunity.

A lack of biotin shows up as painful muscles, can't think right, super sensitive skin, pricking feelings, loss of appetite, sick to stomach, a rash on the arms and legs, down in the dumps, loss of hair, sore tongue, no energy, can't sleep, nervousness, and a grayish skin color. A note of caution, eating many raw egg whites will cause loss of biotin because raw egg white contains avidin which binds with biotin in the intestine and keeps it from being absorbed into the body.

We find biotin in all animal and plant foods, especially in yeast, soybeans, egg yolk, peanut butter, mushrooms, liver, dark green vegetables, brown rice, and whole grains.

CHOLINE

Choline is present in all foods. It is needed to make important parts of all cell membranes and to make a substance needed throughout the body, (acetylcholine). Choline was found in 1862 by Strecker and made chemically in 1866. Without choline, the body develops problems with the liver, kidneys, pancreas, brain (loss of memory), and the body can't grow properly. Over a period of time the liver becomes a fatty liver and cirrhosis (hardening of the liver) occurs. Other results include high blood pressure, heart disease, and hardening of the arteries. The body can make choline from folic acid, B12 and methiomine. We also find choline in lecithin, liver, brewer's yeast, wheat germ, and egg yolk.

INOSITOL

Inositol is found in foods from plants and animals, but the best source is lecithin from egg yolk, or from commercial preparations, often soy based. Inositol can also be synthesized by bacteria in the intestine. It helps nourish the brain cells. It is needed for growth and survival of cells in the bone marrow, eye membranes, and the intestines. The adrenal glands need inositol to do their work. Inositol and choline work together to prevent hardening of the arteries to protect the liver, kidneys, and heart. Inositol and choline work together in keeping us from bleeding too much. Lecithin, a prime source of inositol from egg yolk, can prevent hair thinning and baldness and helps hair grow.

Little babies need a lot of inositol, and breast milk contains a lot of it; the colostrum \which comes out first when the baby starts nursing has an even higher amount. When I delivered babies, I urged the mothers to breast feed their babies even for a little while even if they had to go back to work and had to bottle feed them later.

Large amounts of coffee can wipe out the body's stores of inositol. A lack of inositol shows up in constipation, skin rashes, eye problems, heart disease, hardening of the arteries, hair loss, high blood cholesterol, and the person may become so very thin that he looks like skin and bones. Such a person will need plenty of inositol found in lecithin, liver, brewer's yeast, unprocessed whole grains and cereals, molasses, oranges, lemons, limes, most foods from plants and animals.

PABA (PARA-AMINOBENZOIC ACID)

PABA helps the body make folate (folic acid) which then helps the body make pantothenic acid. PABA and pantothenic acid work together as anti-stress vitamins, also in the health of skin in delaying wrinkles, and in preventing the loss of hair color. PABA acts as a sunscreen and is included in some commercial sunscreens. PABA helps the body use proteins and form blood cells, especially red blood cells. A lack of PABA causes tiredness, out of sorts, down in the dumps, nervousness, headache, constipation, and stomach problems. The friendly bacteria in our intestines can make PABA which is also found in liver, brewer's yeast, yogurt, milk, eggs, whole grains and cereals, wheat germ, brown rice, and molasses.

B15 (PANGAMIC ACID)

B15 is widely used in Russia and other European countries. It helps the body use oxygen and blood sugar. B15 treats a low level of oxygen and thus it is helpful in protecting against the damaging effects of carbon monoxide poisoning. B15 is important in the prevention and treatment of cancer as normal cells need oxygen, but cancer cells thrive without oxygen.

B15 is useful in treating circulation problems whether in the heart, legs, brain, or other parts of the body. It has been used to treat asthma, emphysema, chest pain, premature aging, rheumatism, alcoholism, and high blood cholesterol. B15 helps the body use fat, sugar, and protein and feeds cells all over the body including the heart, glands, and nerves.

Vitamins A and E work with B15. If we don't get enough B15 we don't get enough oxygen to the cells and this damages the heart, glands, nerves, and brain. If the body receives more B15 than needed, the excess is eliminated through the kidneys, bowels and sweat.

Pangamic Acid (B15) was originally found in an extract of apricot kernels and later in crystalline form from other sources. We can get B15 by eating whole grains and cereals, brown rice, rice bran, rice polish, brewer's yeast, pumpkin and sesame seeds.

B17 (LAETRILE, AMYGDALIN, OR NITRILOSIDES)

B17 is an amygdalin, a simple chemical compound consisting of two molecules of sugar, one molecule of benzaldehyde, and one molecule of cyanide. Nitrilosides are known as "laetrile" when used in medical dosage form. Laetrile was first used by a Chinese herbalist, Pen T'Sao in 2800 B.C. and has been in use since that time. It has not received Food and Drug Administration approval in the U.S. It is used legally and is manufactured in many countries throughout the world, including Mexico, Canada, Germany, Italy, Belgium, and the Philippines.

According to the experts, laetrile is a highly selective substance that attacks only cancer cells. When laetrile is eaten and absorbed by normal cells, an enzyme called rhodanese detoxifies the cyanide, which is excreted in the urine. Cancer cells don't have any rhodanese; another enzyme beta-glucosidase releases the cyanide from the laetrile right by the cancer cells, and the cyanide then kills the cancer cells. Laetrile attacks only cancer cells. Laetrile is made from apricot pits. It is found in over 2000 known unrefined foods and grasses. A concentration of about 2 or 3% laetrile is found in the whole kernels of most fruits including apricots, apples, cherries, peaches, plums and nectarine.

VITAMIN C (ASCORBIC ACID)

Vitamin C is soluble in water as are all the B vitamins just described. Human beings along with monkeys and guinea pigs are among the few kinds of animals not able to make Vitamin C from glucose sugar due to lack of a necessary enzyme. Vitamin C was shown to prevent and cure scurvy. It was named ascorbic acid because it was anti-scorbutic (anti-scurvy).

Among diseases connected to nutrition, scurvy is one of the highest in suffering and death. The ancient civilizations of Egypt, Greece and Rome had descriptions of scurvy. Within months of leaving home, the sea explorers of the 16th, 17th and 18th centuries had bleeding and rotting gums, swollen and painful joints, dark blotches on the skin and weak muscles, all symptoms of no vitamin C. Of Admiral Anson's six ships circling the globe in 1740 to 1744 only the flagship returned and 1051 men died. This prompted the British to seek a cure for scurvy. In 1747 Scottish surgeon James Lind tried out 6 different diet additions, and it was proven that oranges and lemons cured scurvy. It was 48 years later that lemon or lime juice was made part of the British Navy rations. British sailors become known as limeys because of the lime juice served to the crew to prevent scurvy.

On land; much of Europe during the great potato famine, the armies of the Crimean wars, both north and south armies of the United States Civil War, arctic explorers and gold rush communities were plagued by scurvy.

We need vitamin C to make collagen, the cement which literally holds our cells together. We also need it to make elastin. We must have vitamin C for broken bones to knit, for surgical wounds, pressure sores, cuts and scratches to heal. A lack of collagen causes the tissues to be loose and watery, allowing bacteria and viruses to travel more easily throughout the body. Vitamin C is needed to make carnitine which is needed for fatty acids stored in our fat cells to be turned into energy. Vitamin C is needed for the muscle of the heart, and for muscles all over our bodies. If we don't have enough vitamin C, we get weak and tired. Vitamin C helps iron be absorbed by getting iron into a more absorbable ferrous rather than ferric form and works with iron in the body including making red blood cells. It help the liver get rid of cholesterol as bile acids in bile. Vitamin C prevents foods and heavy metals from forming cancer-causing substances. Vitamin C is needed to make hormones in the adrenal glands. In the brain vitamin C is used to form a substance which produces happy attitudes.

Vitamin C is absorbed in the intestine and any extra is gotten rid of by the kidneys. The level of vitamin C varies in various parts of our bodies. There is more in the pituitary gland, the adrenals, the white blood cells, lens of the eyes, and brain, and less in the saliva and plasma of the blood.

Vitamin C in white blood cells helps in giving us better immunity against disease. As an anti-oxidant., it protects all our cells from the ravages of free radicals of oxygen, and against aging. Bodily needs for vitamin C increase with stress, infection, illness, injury, physical exercise, pregnancy, nursing a baby, air pollution, surgery, and cigarette smoking. Each cigarette uses up 25mg of Vitamin C, which is 500mg per pack. Lack of vitamin C shows up in tiny and larger hemorrhagic spots, coiled hairs, sore bleeding gums, thickened scaly skin, dry mouth, shortness of breath, swelling of joints and ankles, painful joints, and poor wound healing. Other symptoms include weakness, tired out, weariness, down in the dumps, thinking one has a disease with no evidence for it, unstable widening and narrowing of blood vessels, bleeding into the joints, into the sac around the heart, and into the abdominal cavity. There can be bleeding in the adrenal glands and in the gums.

In infants bones don't grow normally or even grow. There can be hemorrhages behind the eyeballs, nosebleeds, blood in urine, and anemia from blood loss. The baby may not move just because it hurts too much to move, and this can be mistaken for paralysis.

Light, heat and air can destroy vitamin C. That's a good reason to eat the orange and not squeeze it into juice, as the oxygen in the air destroys a lot of its vitamin C in the process of squeezing. Vitamin C can be lost in cooking and in cooking water. There is lots of vitamin C in fresh fruits especially citrus such as oranges, lemons, and limes, and vegetables such as red and green peppers, broccoli, turnip greens, collard greens, parsley, cabbage, cauliflower, and Brussel sprouts. Vitamin pills and capsules are available.

VITAMIN D

Vitamin D is known as the "sunshine vitamin". The sun's ultraviolet rays act on a form of cholesterol in the skin (7 dehydrocholesterol) to make previtamin D3 which becomes vitamin D and gets taken to the liver to be stored. Older people can make only 30% as much as younger people. As vitamin D is needed for healthy bones, it is very important to check to see if there is enough vitamin D to prevent various bone fractures; also enough to prevent the decreased height of back bones which causes older people to be shorter as they age. Usually with young people, being in the sun even 15 minutes a day in the summer is enough to have storage over the winter. The melanin in the skin is a sunscreen, so people with darker skin need more time in the sun. In areas away from the equator more time in the sun is needed, and they may need to take cod liver oil or a capsule containing vitamin D, and the capsule needs to have a hole put in it to be sure that its contents can be absorbed.

As with all vitamins that dissolve in fat, not water, vitamin D capsules need to be taken with or after a meal containing some fat or oil. Vitamin D helps calcium and phosphorus be absorbed from the intestine. After that it is responsible for keeping the amount of calcium inside and outside of cells at the right level. If we don't eat enough calcium and phosphorous, vitamin D takes calcium and phosphorus from our bones and puts them into the blood vessels to take to the cells so that the body can work.

When we don't get enough vitamin D, this results in rickets in children and in osteomalacia in adults. Children's bones and teeth don't develop normally and they don't grow normally and are weak. In osteomalacia adults have pain in their bones, and just touching their bones causes pain. They hurt to move about and don't have the strength to do so. They also break their bones very easily. Fish liver oils such as cod liver oil are the best natural source of vitamin D. In the US vitamin D has been added to milk. Capsules containing vitamin D are sold in stores.

During the 18th and 19th centuries cod liver oil was used as a common folklore medicine for prevention and cure of rickets. In 1827 Bretoneau treated acute rickets in a 15 month old child with cod liver oil and noted how fast the child was cured. His student Trousseau added exposure to sunlight to the use of oils from fish and sea mammals for a rapid cure of rickets. Cod liver oil also contains vitamin A. To show that it wasn't the vitamin A that cured rickets, they heated the cod liver oil with oxygen to get rid of the vitamin A, and then used this oil to cure rickets, and then they realized that they had a new fat-soluble vitamin that was called vitamin D. When northern Europe got a lot of factories, people got less sun. In 1822 Sniadecki noticed that children living in Warsaw had lots of rickets, but children living in the country did not. In 1889 in Britain a study noted that children in the cities had rickets, but not in the Highlands out in the country. In 1921 7 children with rickets were put in the sunshine on the roof of a New York City hospital and later x-rays showed that the rickets was improved; new calcium was formed in the growing parts of bones. Hooray! Our country still has a lot of people who don't have enough vitamin D, even in sunny Florida and California.

VITAMIN E

Vitamin E was first found in wheat germ oil. In 1922 rats were fed food that had enough vitamins A, B, C, and D to keep them healthy and growing well, but they couldn't have baby rats. The missing vitamin was a soluble fat vitamin which prevented the death of the unborn young. By 1925 vitamin E was accepted as the 5th serial alphabetical name for the vitamin. Then Evans proposed the word tocopherol from the Greek "tos" for childbirth and "phero" meaning to bring forth, and "ol" for the alcohol part of the molecule. By 1938 chemists were able to make vitamin E in the lab.

In 1953 a professor in Obstetrics and Gynecology at Ohio State University, Dr. Keys, prescribed wheat germ for his patients who had had problems with miscarriages. In one study, the husbands were given 100 IU of vitamin E daily, and the wives were given 200 IU of vitamin E daily; 100 couples had 79 pregnancies with 77 babies and 2 miscarriages. Before taking vitamin E they had had 144 pregnancies all ending in miscarriages.

Vitamin E works with vitamin C and Selenium to protect cells all over our bodies from the effect of oxygen running loose, much like the browning of a cut apple. They also protect the body from the cancer-causing substances formed from nitrates and nitrites in cured meats such as ham, bacon, and sausage. Vitamin E has been known to relieve or cure over 80 illnesses. It prevents hardening of arteries. Vitamin E helps us heal wounds, burns, surgical scars, cuts, bruises, hurt muscles and tendons. It helps protect the heart and the brain.

A combination of 800 IU of vitamin E and 500mg of vitamin C is recommended to have anti-ageing effect, to improve wound healing and to protect bones from the bad effect of smoking. Vitamin E 1000 IU twice a day has been recommended as a treatment for Alzheimer's disease along with lots of fruits, vegetables, and fish and a healthy lifestyle. This is good for the heart as well as the brain. Vitamin E is stored in the liver and the fatty tissues. Any vitamin E that isn't needed goes out mainly in the bowel movement, very little in the urine. Invite Vitamin E to dinner by having nuts, wheat germ, soy beans, seeds, and vegetable oils.

VITAMIN K

Vitamin K is another vitamin that is soluble in fat. When we get a cut, the reason we don't just keep bleeding is that the vitamin K goes to work to help our blood to clot, and the bleeding stops. Our bones and kidneys need vitamin K, too. Not much is stored in our bodies. We need a daily supply. Our good bacteria in our intestines are able to make some vitamin K.

1929 Henrik Dam in Copenhagen, Denmark was studying sterol metabolism in chicks fed fat-free diets. To his surprise, some chicks got big bruise areas in their skin and muscles. He took some blood samples to the lab and there was a delay in clotting. They found that hemorrhagic disease was due to a lack of prothrombin activity in the plasma of the blood. They found that the vitamin which stopped bleeding was soluble in fat but it was not any of the already known vitamins, vitamin A, B, C, D, or E.

They named it vitamin K for Koagulation (Danish). They found vitamin K in liver, hemp seeds, alfalfa, and green leafy vegetables. In 1939 they made vitamin K from alfalfa. Doisy and staff made vitamin K from rotten fish meal.

A substance that worked opposite to vitamin K was found in spoiled clover in 1941 by Campbell and Link; they called it dicumerol (Warfarin, Coumadin). The spoiled clover had caused a hemorrhagic (bleeding) disease in cattle, noted in 1922 by Schofield.

The forming of the 2 bone proteins which need vitamin K depends on Vitamin D. Vitamin K is sensitive to light. Warfarin keeps the body from making the 2 bone proteins, osteocalcin and matrix Gla protein (MGP). Osteocalcin is like the chicken wire nailed to the side of a house so that the stucco or plaster can grip the surface.

In one study people with osteoporosis (thin porous bones) had only 35% as much vitamin K as a similar group of people who had normal bones. Proteins which depend on vitamin K are also found in kidney, spleen, lung, womb, placenta (afterbirth), pancreas, thyroid, thymus, and testicles; all these also have to do with binding calcium. All 7 of the coagulation proteins need calcium to work.

Bring Vitamin K to the table at breakfast, lunch, and supper with egg yolk, leafy green vegetables, cabbage, broccoli, cauliflower, Brussel sprouts, milk and other dairy products, meats, cereals, fruits, other vegetables. Yogurt and kefir have friendly bacteria which can make vitamin K in the intestine. All fat soluble vitamins including vitamin K need to be taken with fats or oils, for example with nuts or peanut butter. They also need bile and juices form the pancreas to be absorbed. Extra goes out in the urine and the bowel movements.

If vitamin K is missing, nosebleeds, other bleeding such as bruising, splinter hemorrhages under the nails and in the whites of the eyes, other parts of the skin, pale skin, vomiting up blood, blood in the urine and in the bowel movement can give clues to this. Bleeding can occur in any part of the body including the brain, spinal cord, and intestines. New born babies routinely receive a shot of vitamin K.

SIMPLY NUTRITION III, MINERALS CALCIUM

*T*here is more Calcium in our bodies than any other mineral, and 99% of it is in our bones and teeth. But don't think that the other 1% isn't important; we couldn't live without it. Our bodies are made up of cells and every cell must have calcium. Every cell has a covering called membrane, and works on its own, but also works with other cells.

Calcium and phosphorus work together. Vitamin D helps both get into the body from the foods we eat. Bones have 2 ½ times as much calcium as phosphorus. In 1862 Hoppe-Seyler noted that the calcium phosphate in the apatite parts of rocks was like the calcium phosphate in bones and teeth. Apatite is also called hydroxyapatite. Here is a little rock that looks like a green, blue, or yellow stone that is like an important part of our bones and teeth.

The 1% that isn't in bones and teeth does a lot of jobs. It works in the heart to keep it beating right. If we get a cut, it helps the blood to clot. Every time we move our fingers, arms, and legs and for all our muscles to move, calcium is at work helping us. All kinds of chemical messengers, our hormones, our enzymes, our brain signals all need calcium. Extra calcium goes out in bowel movement, a small amount in urine and a tiny amount in sweat.

There are tiny spots on our bones made especially as reception centers for certain hormones. There is one for male hormone, testosterone. There is one for female hormone, estrogen. There is one for growth hormone. If a lady has her menopause and she stops having menstrual periods, she needs to take estrogen for her bones. Men in later years often have a drop in their testosterone, and should be given testosterone for their bones. Older men as well as older ladies often get hip fractures (broken bones). These could be prevented. Vitamin D levels in the blood also need to be checked; D is important in maintaining healthy bones. Magnesium, vitamin A and C also work with calcium.

If the thyroid gland makes too much thyroid hormone, or if the person it taking too much thyroid hormone, calcium is taken out of the bones and the bones get porous (osteoporosis). The bones need just the right amount of thyroid hormone. If the thyroid gland gets too big, usually because of not getting enough iodine, it is called a goiter. Sometimes the thyroid gland needs surgery; then sometimes the 4 tiny parathyroid glands (para=next to) are hurt or accidently taken out. The parathyroid glands make a hormone to keep the calcium just right; calcium in the body can get too low if there is not enough hormone from the parathyroid glands. On the other side of the coin, if the parathyroid glands are making too much parathormone, such as if there is a parathyroid tumor, the calcium level can get too high. In the worst case scenario, very high calcium can make the heart stop beating. A cardiogram (EKG) can tell us if the calcium level is too high or too low or just right while we are waiting for the report from the lab to tell us how much calcium is in the blood.

Look for a low calcium if there is tingling around the mouth, hands, and feet, twitchy muscles, spasms of the bronchi in the lungs, and of the larynx (voice box). Low calcium can cause down in the dumps, can't think right, cataracts, poor development of the enamel of teeth, no energy, and jumpy. Too much calcium can cause low muscle tone, down in the dumps, mixed up mind, feeling blah, even unconsciousness. So let's drink milk or eat other things made from milk. Other foods can give us calcium, too. Eat dark green leafy vegetables, nuts, tofu, maple syrup, seaweeds, soft bones of fish, legumes (beans, lentils, peas), brewer's yeast, black strap molasses, sesame seeds, carob, parsley, watercress, radishes, apples, pears, sardines, salmon, caviar, egg yolks, soybeans, almonds, and Brazil nuts.

PHOSPHORUS

Foods high in protein are also high in phosphorus. Eat meat, poultry, fish, eggs, and milk and some whole grain cereals and there will be plenty of phosphorus. Only people on a very poor diet who take anti-acids that bind up the phosphorus are likely to not have enough phosphorus. Our bones and teeth have 85% of our phosphorus. Our muscles have 14%. The 1% left is spread out in very important places. Phosphorus is in all the membranes which make the walls for all our cells, and in the fluid inside all cells. It is part of all the enzymes that turn food into energy, and do all kinds of other jobs in our bodies.

When large amounts of alcohol are taken into the body, acetate is formed as a result of the body using alcohol for fuel instead of food. The acetate goes into the cell causing the phosphorus to leave the cell. The alcohol acts like a poison to the kidneys and they leak phosphorus because the little kidney tubes are not able to absorb the phosphorus back into the body. This causes a low phosphorus level. The result is poor appetite, weakness, anemia, the white blood cells can't fight infection, the platelets can't help the blood to clot when we get a cut. Breathing is off kilter. Muscles are weak and painful. Damaged nerves are tingly and don't support normal walking and movement. Seizures and unconsciousness may result. The parathyroid glands and pancreas are not able to do their work. The heart muscle and kidneys cannot work normally.

MAGNESIUM

A low amount of magnesium is very common in the United States because processed foods have lost 3/4th of their magnesium. How do we get a good supply of this very important mineral? Magnesium is high in whole grains, wheat germ, nuts, fish, soybeans, legumes such as lentils, beans and peas, and green leafy vegetables. Other good sources include fresh meat, pumpkin seeds, dried fruits, fresh fruits, and black strap molasses (52mg, per tablespoon).

Magnesium is at the center of all energy systems, and is needed for blood sugar (glucose) balance. In one study, 582 diabetic people had a much lower magnesium level in the blood than 140 people who did not have diabetes. Low magnesium shows up as poor appetite, sick to stomach, vomiting, dizziness, weakness, no get-up-and-go, down in the dumps, worried about what might happen, panic attacks, heart beating fast and pounding, can't sleep and tired out.

When I had a patient in Coronary Care Unit (for heart patients) I checked their Magnesium, Calcium, and Phosphorus levels in addition to the 7 survey which checked Sodium, Potassium, Chloride, Blood

Sugar, and other blood chemistries. Magnesium is very important for the heart. Magnesium helps the heart have normal rhythm and helps the blood vessels to relax and not tighten up. Giving magnesium has helped heart patients to live and not die.

The brain needs magnesium; its memory center, the hippocampus, scoops up magnesium like a magnet. A 76 year old man with memory loss (Alzheimer's disease) in a nursing home, not paying attention to things around him, was given 500mg of magnesium twice a day. In 2 or 3 weeks the doctors were surprised to see that he was noticing things around him, and his wife and son were delighted when he called his wife by name, first time in months. He continued to do better and was able to go home in 9 months.

Magnesium relaxes muscles and calms nerves. It relaxes muscles in the bronchial tubes of the lung and can help asthma. It relaxes the muscles in blood vessels in the brain, the heart, the colon, and all over the body, bringing better flow of blood and oxygen to the area. One doctor recommended 800mg of magnesium per day to get the plumbing working again along with plenty of water. Incidentally, Epsom salts has long been used as a remedy for constipation; it is hydrated magnesium sulfate. Epsom salts is named after Epsom a town in Surrey, England, where it was found in a mineral spring. A too high magnesium can happen if someone accidently or on purpose takes too much Epsom salts. This almost never happens. If magnesium is too much in the body, prickling of the face and sleepiness are warning signals. Later breathing is slower or can stop, unconsciousness, decreased reflexes, slowed heart rate and heart can stop beating.

POTASSIUM

Potassium and magnesium play important roles inside our cells. There is 38 times as much potassium inside our cells as there is outside our cells. This amount is needed for our nerves and muscles to work. Sodium and chloride are mainly outside the cells in the fluid around cells. Salt is sodium chloride, a combination of sodium and chloride. So we have a lot of salt water in our bodies. But we don't want too much or we get swollen. The heart is particularly sensitive to the presence of enough potassium and stops beating if the level of potassium gets too low. A lady I know died because the potassium got too low. Too much salt can cause a low potassium. Not enough magnesium can cause a low potassium. As the blood sugar rises after a meal, insulin also rises and works with hormones from the adrenal glands to get potassium into cells including muscle and liver cells. The adrenal glands put out another hormone to keep a proper balance when extra potassium is present. In case of kidney damage, the intestines take over and get rid of extra potassium as needed. Normally our bodies do a great balancing act. However, uncontrolled diabetes with high urine output can lower potassium. Diarrhea, use of too many laxatives, and vomiting can lower potassium, also a lot of sweating. Eating clay (geophagia) binds potassium and iron. Sugar, caffeine and alcohol can cause the body to lose potassium and magnesium. Potassium helps the cells keep the proper amount of water in them.

Normal growth and use of muscles depend on potassium. Potassium is needed to store glucose as glycogen to be used later for energy, and also to make proteins for muscles. When the kidneys cannot put out enough urine, the potassium level can get too high.

EKG changes show up before it even shows up in the blood. If the potassium level gets too high there is weakness, decreased breathing and muscle tone, and later the heart beats fast and irregularly and then stops. In a person who is skin and bones, the lost potassium is replaced by sodium and water in the cells, and the person is weak and very tired. We get lots of potassium when we eat vegetables, fruits, whole grains, potatoes, nuts, meat, fish, eggs, milk and milk products, and sunflower seeds. Citrus fruits such as oranges and lemons, raisins, and bananas are great ways to get potassium.

Sodium and water

Our bodies are about 54% water. Half of this is inside cells and half outside of cells. Water is needed for everything the body does. The body is nourished through waterways in our bodies. Water is part of the urine, part of the bowel movements and part of the sweat to get rid of wastes from the body. Water helps the body keep a normal temperature. The rate of water loss in sweat depends on the amount of activity and the climate or temperature in the house. The part of blood that is not cells, such as red blood cells, white blood cells and platelets, is called plasma. Plasma is 93% water and 7% plasma proteins and lipids (fats and fat-like substances). Sodium is dissolved in plasma water. Sodium controls where the water in the body goes and just how acid or alkaline a body fluid is. We need a certain amount of sodium taken as salt (sodium chloride) to stay healthy. Too much salt causes high blood pressure and osteoporosis (porous bones which break easily). Our ancestors ate only less than 1000mg (1 gram) per day and took in 10 times as much potassium as sodium, whereas today we take in twice as much sodium as potassium. Not over 2400mg is recommend. In the US 4000mg is the usual daily amount eaten. We need to take in at least 115mg and 500mg is advised. There is a good supply of sodium in foods from animals such as meat, poultry, fish, eggs, and milk. We mainly get sodium in salt and seasoning or preservatives added to processed foods. Man has added salt to food for over 3000 years. Sodium is easily absorbed in the small intestine and colon. Kidneys reabsorb the amount of sodium and water needed to get rid of the rest. Low sodium causes giddiness, weakness, a don't care attitude, worn out, cramps, loss of appetite, sick to stomach, vomiting, later headache, decreased awareness, feel dizzy, feel confused and not able to think. If sodium gets low enough there is loss of consciousness and breathing stops. On the other hand, too high a sodium can come from people taking too many salt pills in hot weather or from a loss of water as in a lot of sweating in hot weather, diarrhea, or vomiting. Fever, severe burns, and diuretics (water pills can cause a loss of water. Poorly controlled diabetics lose a lot of water and may develop a high sodium problem. People on ventilators can lose a lot of water. High sodium can cause mental problems, weakness, problems with nerves and muscles, even seizures and loss of consciousness. A decreased brain cell volume from a loss of water can cause hemorrhage in the brain or into the space around the brain.

Chloride

Chloride is joined to sodium to form salt and it works with sodium all through the body. Joined to hydrogen, chloride is in the hydrochloric acid in the stomach, so important in the digestion of food and in releasing B12 from food. Chloride can be lost in vomiting with a loss of stomach acid. If vomiting continues, the blood may become too alkaline due to the loss of acid from the body. Chloride comes into the body along with sodium as salt and both are absorbed together in the intestines.

SULFUR

Sulfur is a pale yellow element present in all proteins. Thus it is in every cell of our bodies. One quarter of 1% of our bodies is sulfur. The amino acids cystine, methionine, and taurine contain sulfur. Chondroitin sulfate is the main ground substance of cartilage, bone, blood vessels, and other connective tissues of the body. Sulfur is needed to make collagen. Sulfur is a part of keratin, a tough protein substance in skin, nails, and hair. Insulin and heparin contain sulfur. The B vitamins B1 (thiamine), and biotin contain sulfur.

Sulfur is part of some enzyme systems. It is needed to transfer energy. Sulfur is used to remove toxins and poisons. It works with the liver to put out bile. Sulfur, though present in every cell of the body, is highest in hair, skin, and nails. Our kidneys and our digestive tract get rid of any sulfur we don't need. Many foods are good sources of sulfur, especially meat, fish, poultry, eggs, milk products, soybeans, nuts, legumes such as lentils and beans. Other foods contain sulfur including fruits, vegetables, onions, garlic, horseradish, chives, red hot peppers, potatoes, sesame, pumpkin and sunflower seeds.

TRACE ELEMENTS

IRON

Swords and spears and axes were made from iron by people a long time ago. When iron is left out and gets wet, unless it is stainless steel (iron with other materials added to it), it gets rusty. In the Ebers papyrus of Egypt, the oldest manuscript we have, it is recorded that rust was put into an ointment and used to prevent baldness. In ancient Greece, iron was dissolved in wine and given to men to restore their ability to father children. In 1895 Stockman showed that young women with anemia had diets low in iron compared to persons who were normal. In 1932 Health showed that giving iron to people with anemia due to lack of iron, corrected the anemia.

Hemoglobin in the red blood cells carries the oxygen from the lungs to all parts of our bodies. The hemoglobin is made up of 3.8% heme and 96.2% globin. The globin is the protein part and the heme is the part that gives the red blood cell its red color and carries the oxygen. The heme contains iron. Hemoglobin has 4 heme groups (containing iron) to each globin group (containing proteins).

Myoglobin, (hemoglobin of muscle) has 1 heme group to each globin group, and the heme part carries the oxygen; it picks up the oxygen from the hemoglobin in the blood and allows it to transfer to the muscle which needs it for energy to move the muscle. Carbon dioxide (CO_2) is the byproduct and the heme in hemoglobin (in the tiny little blood vessels in the muscle called capillaries) picks up the CO_2 and off goes the little truck on its journey back to the lungs where we breathe out the CO_2. A new supply of oxygen hops on the hemoglobin to be taken to all parts of our bodies. Take a deep breath and breathe in the good air and breathe out the bad air.

When hemoglobin is exposed to carbon monoxide, the oxygen is moved out and the carbon monoxide moves in to stay as the fairly stable carboxylhemoglobin bent on doing long time damage all over the body.

How do we get this iron to make our hemoglobin? Meat, liver, lamb, egg yolk, and dark meat of chicken and turkey are great sources from animals. Vegetable sources are beans, peas, nuts and seeds, and green leafy vegetables. The iron from animals contains heme and is easiest for our bodies to use.

The iron must be absorbed (taken up like a sponge takes up water) in our intestines, and this is better if acid is present from the stomach. Vitamin C also helps the body absorb iron by changing it to the form easier to absorb (ferric to ferrous). Selenium and vitamin E also help in this process. Our bodies are very clever at holding on to the iron by recycling it into new red blood cells as the old ones are gobbled up by special cells in the liver and spleen. More than 90% of hemoglobin iron is recycled again and again. Usually only a tiny amount of iron is lost to the body each day in waste from the intestines, urine, sweat, hair and shed skin cells. About two thirds of the body's iron is in the hemoglobin of red blood cells in our blood. Some is in myoglobin in muscles. Most of the rest of it is stored in the liver, spleen, and bone marrow.

How common is lack of enough iron? One third of the women in the US don't have enough iron. It is most common in women who can have children (39%). It is also common in young children. All over the world anemia is common and causes poor health. When I was a teenager, my mom was so tired and the doctor found out that she was anemic and put her on iron pills and told her to eat liver every day. Other symptoms of anemia are weakness, shortness of breath, pale skin, fast heartbeat, feeling cold, and brain seems fuzzy. If iron is very low fingernails get a spoon shape, mouth is sore and it is hard to swallow. Children don't grow in height and weight as much as they should, and they can't do as well in school and may have behavior problems. The immune system is affected if the iron is low, and people are more likely to get colds and flu. Many enzymes, even those that do not contain iron, are affected by a lack of iron and do not work as well. This includes monoamine oxidase (MAO), a copper-containing enzyme important in making neurotransmitters (important messengers in the brain to carry signals) and platelets for clotting of blood.

COPPER

About 400 BC Hippocrates, a Greek doctor, gave substances containing copper to people to cure lung diseases and other diseases. In the late 19th century, copper was found in the blood. By 1900 animals on a whole milk diet were found to have an anemia which couldn't be prevented by giving iron alone. In 1928 Hart found that he had to give copper as well as iron to anemic rats to cure their anemia. Copper takes part in at least 15 enzyme systems, affecting immunity and in making collagen, elastin, and neurotransmitters (nerve messengers in the brain). Monoamine oxidase (MAO), a copper-containing protein, is involved in many body processes including products of the adrenal gland, and nerve messengers in the brain such as serotonin, norepinephrine, tyramine, and dopamine.

We need copper to make bone, blood vessels, skin, lungs, teeth, cartilage, tendons, ligaments, cornea, and discs between vertebrae. Copper is important in the soundness of the structure of the connective tissue of the heart. Copper plays an important part in the making of hemoglobin. That is the reason why we must have copper as well as iron to treat anemia. Copper is part of a lot of enzymes and is involved in so many body processes.

We could not live without copper. One example is the loss of color in the skin and hair when there is not enough copper. Lack of copper in poorly nourished children shows up as anemia, a low white blood cell count, and soft bones without minerals to keep them strong. A mild lack of copper over a long period of time may show up as arthritis, disease of arteries, heart disease, loss of color of skin and hair, and problems with nerves. Some of the copper is absorbed in the stomach but most in the intestines. Copper not needed goes out in bile which then goes into the intestine and out in the bowel movement. Only small amounts go out in urine, sweat, and shed dead skin.

So how do we get the copper we need? Eat liver, brewer's yeast, seafood, green leafy vegetables, nuts, seeds, cocoa powder, lentils, dried beans, peas and other legumes, whole grains, raisins, prunes, kidney, broccoli, and mushrooms.

ZINC

Men have known for years that oysters give a boost to their sex life. Three ounces of oysters supply 28mg of zinc, and zinc is very important to that area of life. Don't worry if you don't have a ready supply of oysters. Other shellfish (except shrimp), meat, liver, blackstrap molasses, brewer's yeast, wheat germ, whole grains, sesame seeds, pumpkin seeds, maple syrup, legume such as lentils, beans, and peas, and green leafy vegetables will give you the zinc you need to be flying high. Less than a third of adults get enough zinc in what they eat. The other over two thirds don't get enough. Is it any wonder that Viagra is so popular despite its high cost? Dwarfs in Persia and Egypt didn't have normal sexual development and they were found to be low in zinc; this study was in 1961. Zinc had been known since 1509, found to be needed by plants in 1869 and needed by animals in 1934.

Over 95% of our zinc is inside cells, mainly bone cells, but it is in all cells; the other 5% is outside of cells in fluids. Cells can't be made without zinc. Over 200 enzyme systems depend on zinc. Zinc helps our bodies make the collagen which glues us together. We need zinc to have good immunity and not get infections or cancer. Low zinc, and we can't taste or smell. Zinc is needed for us to make growth hormone, hormones from the pituitary gland to hormones made by the ovaries, testicles, thyroid, and adrenal glands; also insulin and prostaglandins (substances made of fatty acids and acting like hormones).

More zinc is needed by diabetics and other conditions which increase need such as in ladies who are pregnant or nursing a baby. Zinc is a natural antihistamine without side effects. As with most minerals, zinc is absorbed in the intestine. Extra zinc leaves the body in bowel movement, a little in urine as most is absorbed back, and a tiny amount in sweat, old dead skin, and shed hair.

What clues do we have that we need more zinc? We feel irritable, like doing nothing, down in the dumps, may not walk straight, have shaky hands and speech slurred. Other clues may be delayed growth and sexual development in children, inability to have sex, low sperm count, loss of hair, skin problems, sore tongue, poor immunity to infections, unhappiness, poorly formed nails, can't see in the dark, slow healing of cuts and burns, poor appetite, and disease of the cornea of the eye (the cornea has the highest zinc concentration in the body). Vitamin A needs zinc to work. If any of these clues show up, on with the zinc.

COBALT

B12 contains cobalt which gives B12 its name, Cobalamin. B12 can be stored in liver up to 30 years. The only toxicity known occurred in heavy drinkers of beer containing cobalt chloride, added to improve foaming. Toxicity showed up as damage to the heart muscle, heart failure, fluid around the heart, bigger size to the thyroid gland, too many red blood cells, and problems in the nervous system. Cobalt is a hard, brittle metallic element. Cobalt salts are used for blue glass and ceramic pigments. Cobalt irradiation units are used in radiation oncology to treat cancer. We can get cobalt in seafood, oysters, clams, meat, kidney, liver, and milk.

MOLYBDENUM

Studies in rats and chickens in 1953 showed that they needed molybdenum for normal growth. Molybdenum is part of a number of enzyme systems which affect the use of uric acid, fluoride, copper, and sulfur in our bodies. It is needed for steroid hormones to work. It is absorbed in the stomach and small intestine. Most of it goes to the liver and kidney which also get rid of any not needed in bile and urine. Normally there is no lack of molybdenum. We get it when we eat whole grains, milk products, liver, kidney, yeast, legumes, and dark green leafy vegetables.

SELENIUM

One Brazil nut eaten daily gives you all the selenium you need, 120mg per nut, over 1 ½ times as much for men and over 2 times as much for women. Seafood, meat, chicken, egg yolk, milk, onions, tomatoes, broccoli, wheat germ, and whole grains give us an ample supply of selenium. Any extra selenium is gotten rid of by the kidneys.

In 1979 we found out how important selenium is to us. Selenium is needed to make thyroid hormone. Selenium works with vitamins A, C, and E to protect our bodies from oxygen running loose as "free radicals," which cause a lot of damage by hardening arteries; contributing to aging and cancers. Thus selenium helps prevent heart attacks, poor circulation to legs, brain, heart, genital organs, and all over the body.

In two areas of China the soil is low in selenium. Keshan Disease in Keshan Province of China is a cardiomyopathy in which the heart muscle is damaged, and there is enlargement of the heart, abnormal rhythm and shock due to the heart. The other disease is Kashin-Beck syndrome with inflammatory arthritis.

MANGANESE

Manganese was found in animal tissues in 1913, and found necessary for animals to grow and to have baby animals in 1931. Most manganese is in bone, liver and the pituitary gland. The mitochondria of cells that do the main work of cells contain a good amount of manganese. It works in making much of our tissues, in making urea and in energy release. Our bodies need manganese to use choline, biotin, vitamins B1 and C. Manganese is needed to make fatty acids, cholesterol (we make 800 mg daily), urea, protein, carbohydrates, and fat. Nursing mothers need it to make milk.

Diabetics were found to have only half as much manganese as non-diabetics. Lack of manganese shows up in a poor tolerance to glucose sugar, dizziness, hearing loss, weight loss, skin problems, nausea and vomiting, loss of hair color, slow growth of hair, bleeding tendencies, and muscles not working together properly. It is absorbed in the small intestine and goes out in the bowel movement. Only a tiny amount goes out in urine.

Bring manganese to the dinner table with nuts, seeds, whole grains, wheat germ, shellfish, coffee, tea, green leafy vegetables, other vegetables such as green beans, squash, cucumbers, pineapple and other fruits.

Iodine

In 1885 Bauman discovered iodine in the thyroid gland. Later David Marine showed that a lack of iodine caused goiter (enlarged thyroid gland). In 1922 Marine and Kimball showed that goiter could be prevented by giving a small amount of iodine to school children in Akron, Ohio. Almost all the body's iodine is in thyroid hormones. Lack of iodine is the most common cause of low thyroid hormone.

When a pregnant woman doesn't have enough iodine, her baby could be a cretin, which is a baby with low iodine. The cretin is small, slow to develop, very slow learner, has thick skin, swollen face, big tongue sticking out, a big belly, and can't hear or talk. Very sad. Low iodine in children causes poor teeth growth and teeth are crooked. Low iodine also causes being tired, don't care attitude, slow heart rate, goiter (enlarged thyroid gland), weight gain, and no energy.

Switzerland was the first to add iodine to salt in 1920. We have iodine added to salt in the US. Here and in most countries with cooler climate potassium iodide is added. In hot humid countries potassium iodate is added because it is not likely to turn into a gas and evaporate. In Thailand in 1980 potassium iodate was added to salt and in 6 years the lack of iodine in school children was lowered from 84% to zero. Just half a gram of the potassium iodide or potassium iodate form of iodine added to a kilogram (1000 grams) of salt does the job.

Although iodized salt is the most common way of getting iodine, foods such as Swiss chard, turnip greens, fish, seafood, and sea vegetables such as kelp supply iodine, too. But there is a warning not to take too much kelp or other sea vegetables, as too much is not good, either. In areas where it is not practical to get salt iodized, giving shots of oil containing iodine have been shown to last over 4 years.

CHROMIUM

In many countries including the US many people eat refined foods such as white flour, white rice and sugar. These refined foods have lost a good deal of their chromium. At the same time many more people have diabetes. When we eat, everything is turned into glucose sugar to be used for energy. Chromium is needed for us to use the glucose sugar in our blood and bodies. It has been estimated that ¼ to ½ the people in the US don't have enough chromium. When people have more stress such as infections, getting hurt or bruised or eat diets high in sugar they need more chromium. A lack of chromium shows up in people becoming diabetic or pre-diabetic, in problems with nerves in feet and hands, and brain problems. Chromium was found in plants and animals in 1948, and in 1959 it was shown to be needed for the body to use sugar. By 1977 it was noted that human beings had to have it. Chromium has to be present for insulin to latch on to spots in the body where it goes to work. Chromium also works with the use of fats, oils, cholesterol, and fatty acids in our bodies. Some enzymes and hormones contain chromium. It is absorbed in the intestine, and extra is gotten rid of mainly in the urine plus small amount in hair, sweat, and bile.

FLUORIDE

Fluoride is made up of fluorine, as gas and another element. It was noticed that there was less tooth decay and stronger heavier bones in areas where there was more fluoride in the soil (dirt) and water. Fluorine in the fluoride stops the enzyme enolase from helping foods such as meat and potatoes change to glucose sugar. Germs which attack the teeth thrive and grow on glucose sugar.

Now many cities have added a wee bit, 1 part per million, to the water supply. In 1945 Grand Rapids, Michigan, was the first city in the world to do this. In Kizileaoern, Turkey, the water has over 5 times as much fluoride, and a traveler to that area noted people in their 30's hobbling about like a very old persons. As toddlers tend to swallow some of their toothpaste, parents need to supervise closely or to use Tom's Natural Toothpaste or Toddler's Toothpaste which contain no fluoride for the children.

Fluoride is found in many foods, but in very small amounts. Fish, Tea, most animal foods, and green vegetables contain fluoride, depending on what is in the water and soil.

SILICON

Silicon helps us have healthy skin, hair and nails. It helps us get calcium and phosphorus into our bodies. Every part of the body has a little silicon in it. In 1848 it was found in the ash left when animals were burned up. Proof that chickens and rats just had to have it was shown in 1972; without it chicks has lopsided skulls and really skinny leg bones. Collagen (gristle) is mostly made up of silicon. Collagen makes up our noses, voice boxes, ears and is in joints and all over our bodies. Silicon is in tendons and eyes. Although a trace mineral, we indeed do need it. We can get it in the herb, horsetail. We can eat it in oats, brown rice, barley, green and red peppers, leafy green vegetables, potatoes with skins, cucumbers with peels, and bean sprouts. Sand is silicon dioxide, but no one eats that on purpose.

NICKEL

Nickel does some of its work with nucleic acid which works with chromosomes. Our bodies have 46 chromosomes, 23 pairs; one of each pair from mother and one of each from father. Females provide xx chromosomes; males provide xy, which determines the sex of the child. Females can give only x to the baby; if males give an x the baby is a girl; if a y chromosome from the male the baby is a boy. Other chromosomes have to do with color of eyes and hair and how tall or short we are and lots of other things. Nucleic acid is also part of the nucleoli, mitochondria, and cytoplasm (fluid in the cell) of all cells. In other words, it is part of the workings of all cells. Although only a tiny amount in the body, it is of great importance.

Nickel also works in some enzyme systems. The thyroid and adrenal glands have a high amount of nickel. Most of any extra nickel we absorb goes out in urine, some in sweat and bile. We can get nickel by eating chocolate, nuts, dried beans and peas, whole grains and cereals, and vegetables.

BORON

Boron helps us get minerals such as calcium into our bones. It works with calcium and estrogen. When boron was increased from 0.25mg to 3.25mg per day, the loss of calcium, phosphorus, and magnesium in urine dropped, and the blood serum level of estradiol (estrogen) increased (1987) report. Our brains need boron. People who had low levels of boron did not do as well as those on higher levels of boron in tests of memory, paying attention, and noticing things. Electroencephalograms showed decreased mental alertness in those with less boron. Extra goes out mainly in urine. Bones, spleen and thyroid have the highest amount of boron. How do we get it? Beans, nuts, vegetables, and fruit such as apples and pears supply us with boron.

ARSENIC

Too much arsenic will kill you. There is a play called "Arsenic and Old Lace"; in it a crazy old lady gave arsenic to men whom she thought it was doing them a favor to kill them. Her "nephew" turned out to be adopted; oh, was he happy to find that out. Fortunately we can't get too much from foods. Seafood is our best source of arsenic. We need arsenic in all our body parts, but the highest amounts are in skin, hair and nails. Arsenic enters the body through the intestines, and extra exits mainly through the urine and minor amounts through bile, sweat, loss of hair and shed skin.

TIN

Tin is found in most parts of our bodies, but none is found in the brain. Maybe that is why the Tin Man in the Wizard of Oz needed a brain. A study on rats in 1990 showed that rats that didn't get enough tin didn't grow as well, had hair loss, and didn't move normally when they heard a noise. Tiny amounts of tin are found in most foods.

VANADIUM

Vanadium has been shown to be a mineral we need even though it is in tiny amounts. Studies since 1987 have backed this up. Vanadium is found throughout our bodies, but is highest in serum (watery part of blood), bones, teeth, and fat. Bones have a lion's share. Important enzyme systems use vanadium. Any excess of vanadium we absorb goes out in the urine. Goats who lacked vanadium had miscarriages and a high death rate of baby goats. They also made less milk. Baby goats had poorly formed lower legs and feet and low thyroid. People seem to get enough vanadium. Foods rich in vanadium include shellfish, fish, mushrooms, parsley, dill seed and other spices. Some is found in fresh fruits and vegetables.

SIMPLY NUTRITION IV, FOODS

Common Sense About Nutrition Sources in Foods (or, What's really in a Bite)

*F*oods contain proteins, carbohydrates, fats and oils, fiber. They also contain vitamins and minerals which are discussed in a separate section.

PROTEIN FOODS: 4 CALORIES PER GRAM

(Calorie, as used here, is a unit of measure of the energy value of food; gram is a unit of weight. Recommended calories per type of food are listed in a separate section.)

Eating protein 3 or more times a day keep the energy coming. No slumps.

Complete Proteins: Meat Poultry Fish Other seafood Eggs Milk Cheese Soybeans

Combined incomplete proteins to produce a combination with all needed amino acid parts equal to a complete protein: 100% Whole Wheat Bread or other Whole-Grain Bread or Crackers, (such as WASA rye crackers), combined with Peanut Butter or Almond Butter, Oatmeal with Walnuts, Split Pea Soup or Lentil Soup with Brown Rice or Barley, Corn Bread and Soup Beans, Brown Rice and Beans, Snack of Miniature Shredded Wheat and Pecans, Peanuts, Almonds, or other Nuts, Popcorn and Peanuts

CARBOHYDRATE FOODS: 4 CALORIES PER GRAM

Health-giving sweets: Raisins Dates Date Sugar Figs Pure Maple Syrup Honey Stevia Black Strap Molasses Dark Molasses Sorghum Other Dried Fruits Grape Juice Apple Juice Pineapple Juice

Whole grains: Oats Brown Rice 100% Whole Wheat Spelt Quinoa Rye Buckwheat Corn Barley Wild Rice Millet used in breads, pancakes, muffins, spaghetti, lasagna, macaroni, and other pastas; and in cakes, cookies, pies, pizza crusts, corn bread, and in soups and stews

VEGETABLES

Minimal calories (almost none): Parsley Bamboo shoots Bean Sprouts Alfalfa Sprouts Bamboo Sprouts and other Sprouts Watercress Salad Greens Garlic Water Chestnuts

Under 10 calories per ½ cup: Lettuce Celery Cucumbers Radishes Zucchini Summer Squash

25 calories per ½ cup: Mushrooms Cabbage Cauliflower Broccoli Green Beans Beets and beet Greens Turnip Greens Mustard Greens Collards Kale Dandelion Greens Spinach Asparagus Green, Red, and Yellow Peppers Pimento Hot Peppers Carrots Eggplant Okra Onions Tomato Rutabaga

Higher calorie vegetables: Corn White Potatoes Sweet Potatoes Yams Winter Squash Acorn Squash Butternut Squash Peas Lentils Lima Beans Died Beans Avocado

FRUITS

Minimal calories: Melons Berries Rhubarb Cranberries

Under 50 to 60 calories: ½ Apple 2 Apricots ½ Banana ½ Grapefruit 10 Grapes 1 Tangerine 1 Clementine ½ Orange 1 Peach 2 Plums or Prunes 10 Cherries ½ Cantaloupe

FATS AND OILS: 9 CALORIES PER GRAM

Oils: Olive, Canola and other non-Hydrogenated Oils. Nuts and Nut Butters (not hydrogenated) are about 50% oil. 1 tablespoon of oil or 2 tablespoons of nuts or nut butters supply the Essential Fatty Acids (EFA's) our bodies need each day. Avocado is one third vegetable oil. Other EFA sources include flaxseed, salmon, mackerel, sardines, anchovies, and herring.

Fats: Butter, Cream and Chicken Fat are good fats. Avoid Margarine, Vegetable Shortening such as Crisco, Hydrogenated Peanut Butters, and many packaged goods (read label).

Percentage of calories in foods which come from the fat in the foods: butter, oil and solid fats, 100%; cream cheese, 87%; sausage, 87%; frankfurters, 82%; bologna, 82%; crisp bacon, 77%; cheddar cheese, 73%; Neufchatel cheese, 71%; well-cooked ground beef, 58%; mozzarella cheese, 56%; low fat (1%) cottage cheese, 11%.

Milk, unless skim, contains protein, carbohydrate, and fat. Protein, 8 grams (32 calories) per cup; Carbohydrate, (as milk sugar, lactose), 12 grams (48 calories) per cup; Fat, whole milk 4%-10 grams (90 calories) per cup; 2% milk – 5 grams (45 calories) per cup; 1% milk – 2.5 grams (22.5 calories) per cup; skim milk – 9 grams (0 calories).

FIBER

Find high fiber in Whole Grains, Beans, Legumes, Vegetables, and Fruit.

HEALTHFUL HINTS

Avoid toxins and robbers of vitamins and minerals such as refined sugars and high fructose corn syrup, refined grains such as white flour and white rice, alcohol and tobacco. There are 8 teaspoons of sugar in 12 oz. of Cola, 1 cup of chocolate milk, 1 cup of sugar-coated cereal, 1 cinnamon roll, 1 piece of Angel Food Cake, 1 pudding, 1 cup ice cream, 2 baking powder biscuits, ½ piece of apple pie, 2 oz. milk chocolate, 2 Brownies, 2 Tbsp. pancake syrup, or 2 rolls. Whole grains and healthful sweets can be substituted in all these, and you can have your cake and eat it, too. Such things trigger an insulin surge which turns these calories into fat cells.

Keep your self hydrated, take in 2 to 3 quarts of water daily. This may be modified in cases of stress on the heart and the urinary system.

Stay active. Walking, riding bike, skating, swimming, skiing, gardening, marketing, baseball, basketball, canoeing, rowing, housework, washing the car, food preparation, golf, tennis are all great.

Think positive thoughts about beautiful and good things. Cheerful attitudes release hormones which enable much health producing activity in the body.

SIMPLY NUTRITION V, RECIPES

OMELET

In a cold skillet put 1 Tbsp. of olive oil. Add 1 onion and 1 bell pepper, cut into bite-sized pieces. Heat skilled to medium heat and cook onion and bell pepper until tender. Beat 6 eggs with ¼ cup of milk, ¼ tsp. Worcestershire sauce, a little black pepper and herb seasoning and add to skillet. Cover. When almost done, sprinkle with shredded Mozzarella cheese and shredded Cheddar cheese. When done serve with toasted or warmed whole wheat or other whole–grain bread or muffins or crackers or grits as desired. Sliced tomatoes is nice, too. Tomato is also nice put into the omelet or scrambled eggs. There are lots of ways of fixing eggs.

OATMEAL

To 6½ cups boiling water add 2 cups oats, and ½ cup each of TVP (texturized vegetable protein) which is soy, and wheat germ. Cook 10 min. Add ½ cup each walnuts and Lecithin Granules. If preferred, just cook the oats in water and serve with nuts, raisins, or other dried and fresh fruits added on top of a bowl of oats.

TUNA MELT

Place a generous amount of tuna on a slice of toasted whole wheat or other whole-grain bread. Cover it with a slice of cheese or shredded cheese. Place under broiler or in a microwave until cheese is melted. Cheddar cheese would be nice. Alternately place tuna melt in a buttered or oiled heavy skillet. Cover. Heat until cheese is melted.

SPLIT PEA SOUP A

Simmer 1 cup of split green peas in 5 cups of water. In a skillet put 1 Tbsp. olive oil. Add ½ cup chopped onion, ½ cup chopped celery with leaves, 3/8 cup sliced carrot, and 1 clove minced garlic. Turn on the heat to medium and cook until soft and add to peas. Add 1 Tbsp. snipped parsley or 1 tsp. dried parsley, ½ tsp. thyme, ½ tsp savory, 1 bay leaf, 2 Tbsp. soy sauce , and ¼ tsp. salt. Total cooking time should be at least 45 min.

SPLIT PEA SOUP B

Simmer 1 cup split green peas and ¼ cup of brown rice or barley in 7 cups of water. Proceed otherwise as in above recipe. Using the green peas with a whole grain such as brown rice or barley then supplies all of the amino acids needed to make a complete protein equivalent to eggs, fish, or meat. Total cooking time should be at least 45 min.

TURKEY SAUSAGE

Mix 1½ tsp. poultry seasoning with 1 lb. of ground turkey. This can be made into patties to serve as such or in hamburger buns (whole wheat or other whole grain buns, bread or crackers). Tiny pieces of it can be cooked and put on top of pizzas. If desired black pepper can be added.

SALMON OR MACKEREL CAKES

Combine 1½ cups of drained canned salmon or mackerel (contents of 1 can) with scant cup of whole wheat or other whole-grain bread crumbs (1 slice), 2 eggs, and 1/8 tsp. paprika. Make into patties and brown on both sides in a little oil. Good with baked potato and cooked carrots. A sauce of cream of mushroom soup or tomato sauce is good with it if desired.

NUT CAKES

Mix 1 cup of ground pecans with 1 tsp. Chile powder, ¼ tsp garlic powder, 1 cup cooked brown rice, 1 cup shredded Mozzarella cheese, 3/8 cup chopped onion, 1 tsp. Worcestershire sauce, and 3 large eggs. Drop by ¼ cup measure on medium hot skillet with a little oil. Flatten slightly. Brown cakes on both sides.

MACARONI AND CHEESE

Cook 2 cups of whole wheat or other whole-grain macaroni in boiling water for 12 min. Melt 2 Tbsp. butter in a saucepan. Add 2 Tbsp. whole wheat or other whole-grain flour. Stir. Add 2 cups milk, ½ tsp. salt, and 1/8 tsp. black pepper. Stir until it thickens. Place alternate layers of cooked macaroni and shredded Cheddar cheese (total of 8 oz.) in a buttered baking dish, ending with cheese. Butter 1 slice of whole wheat or other whole-grain bread and cut it into small cubes; scatter these on top of the macaroni and cheese. Pour sauce over this. Bake at 350 degrees F. for 30 min. until bubbly.

MACARONI AND CHEESE (ALTERNATE RECIPE)

Cook 2 cups (1/2 lbs.) of whole wheat or other whole-grain macaroni in boiling water for 12 min. Combine 1 ½ cups milk, 3 eggs, ½ tsp. salt, ¼ tsp paprika, a dash of cayenne, 4 tsp. dried parsley and beat with a whisk or fork. Place alternate layers of cooked macaroni and shredded Cheddar cheese (total of 8 oz.) in a buttered baking dish, ending with cheese. Pour sauce over this. Butter 1 slice of whole wheat or other whole-grain bread and cut into small cubes;

scatter these on top of the macaroni and cheese. Bake at 360 degrees F for 60 min. or until set. If on a wheat-free or gluten-free diet, brown rice and quinoa pasta is available.

LENTIL DISH

Combine 2 c. cooked lentils, a 14.5 oz. can of diced tomatoes with tomato juice, 1/3 c. of precooked (instant) brown rice or 2/3 c. cooked brown rice, 1 Tbsp. dried green pepper or ¼ c. diced fresh green pepper, 1 tsp. onion powder of ¼ c. diced fresh onion, 1 Tbsp. savory, 1/8 tsp. black pepper, and 1 tsp. cumin. Cook for 15 min.

LENTILS WITH VEGETABLES

Put 1½ cups of washed lentils and 6 cups of water in a 3 quart pot; add 1 Tbsp. cumin, ¾ tsp. salt, and ¼ tsp. pepper. Simmer about 20 min. Cook 1 large sliced onion, 1 diced green pepper, 3 sliced carrots, and ¼ cup snipped parsley (or 4 tsp. dried parsley) in a little oil in a skillet on medium heat till soft and add to lentils. Cook another 15 min.

CHILE CON CARNE

Wash 1 lb. (2 cups) dried pinto or kidney beans. Soak in pot with 6 cups water overnight or for 6 to 8 hours. Simmer 2 hrs. Put 1 chicken bouillon cube into the liquid. Cook 1 chopped onion, 1 chopped green pepper, 1 sliced carrot, and 2 cloves of minced garlic in a little oil in a skillet on medium heat until soft. Add 1 lb. thawed ground turkey or chopped beef and cook until done. Add to cooking beans along with 43.5 oz. of canned tomatoes or tomato puree or chopped tomatoes. Add 2 Tbsp. Chile powder, 1 tsp. paprika, 1 tsp. oregano, ½ tsp. cumin, 1 tsp. basil, ½ tsp. thyme, 1/8 tsp. pepper, 1 bay leaf, and 1 Tbsp. black strap molasses. Simmer 30-60 min. Serve over cooked brown rice. Sprinkle with shredded Cheddar cheese if desired.

GREEN BEAN CHILE

Cook 1 lb. ground beef or turkey with 1 chopped onion. Add 1 can of tomatoes, 1 can of French-cut green beans, 1 small can of V-8 juice, and 2 Tbsp. Chile powder. Simmer for 45 min.

CHICKEN OR TURKEY CURRY

Cook 1 bell pepper and 1 onion cut into bite sized pieces and 1 or 2 sliced stalks of celery in a little oil in a skillet on medium heat. Add 1 lb. of thawed ground turkey or 1 or 2 cups of cooked chicken or turkey cut into bite sized pieces. After browned add 2 apples cut in pieces, ½ cup raisins, 1 Tbsp. curry powder, ½ tsp. ginger, ½ tsp. turmeric, ½ tsp. cumin, and 1 Tbsp. whole wheat or other whole-grain flour. Stir. Add 1 chicken bouillon cube dissolved in 1 cup of hot water and 1 Tbsp. lemon juice. Stir and cook a short time. Serve over cooked brown rice. If desired, sprinkle each serving with almonds.

SPAGHETTI SAUCE

Cook 1 chopped green pepper, 1 chopped onion, and 1 clove minced garlic in a little oil in a skillet on medium heat. Add 1 lb.

thawed ground beef or ground turkey and cook until done. Add 26 oz. of no sugar added spaghetti sauce and 14.5 oz. diced tomatoes in tomato juice. Add 1½ tsp. Italian seasoning, ½ tsp. oregano, ½ tsp basil, 1/16 tsp black pepper and 1 Tbsp. maple syrup or honey. Heat until boiling. Serve over whole wheat, brown rice or quinoa spaghetti. If desired sprinkle with grated Parmesan cheese and shredded Mozzarella cheese.

LASAGNA

In a baking dish place a layer of cooked whole wheat or other whole-grain lasagna, then a layer of spaghetti sauce, then a layer of ricotta or cottage cheese, then a layer of grated Parmesan and shredded Mozzarella cheeses. Repeat layers as needed. Heat in 350 degree F oven until bubbly.

PIZZA

Spread spaghetti sauce thickly over whole wheat Pita bread or on a whole wheat pizza crust. Sprinkle with a thick layer of shredded Mozzarella cheese and some grated Parmesan cheese. Heat in oven or microwave or covered skillet until cheese is melted. If on a wheat-free or gluten-free diet, other whole grain items can be substituted. WASA whole rye crackers are great for those avoiding wheat.

FISH IN MILK-BASED SAUCE

Melt 4 Tbsp. butter (1/4 cup) in a pot. Add ¼ cup whole wheat or other whole grain flour to the butter and mix. Keep heat on low to medium and gradually add 2 cups of milk while stirring. Continue to stir intermittently until mixture thickens and comes to a slow boil. Add about ¼ cup finely chopped onion and about ¼ cup finely chopped green pepper and 1 tsp. Worcestershire sauce. Add 3 cups of cooked fish cut into small pieces. Stir. Sprinkle with black pepper and about ¼ cup of dried parsley. Stir well. Heat to a bubbling boil. Add some boiling water as needed to thin to a good consistency. Serve. Vegetables including potatoes are good accompaniments. Peas and cooked sliced zucchini and summer squash are also good. A raw apple makes a good dessert.

TUNA WITH TOMATO SAUCE AND PASTA

Cook 1 or 2 green peppers and 1 or 2 onions cut in pieces in a little oil in a skilled on medium heat. Add 26 oz. spaghetti sauce and 15 oz. (3 5 oz. cans) tuna fish and 1 tsp. Worcestershire sauce. Serve over whole wheat or other whole-grain pasta, such as penne or spaghetti.

TUNA, RICE AND VEGETABLES

Cook ½ onion, ½ red bell pepper, ½ yellow bell pepper cut into bite-sized pieces, ½ carrot sliced, and 1 stalk celery sliced in a little oil in a skillet on medium heat until soft. Add 1 Tbsp. parsley, a 5 oz. can of tuna, 1 cup cooked brown rice, 1 cup frozen peas, 1 tsp. Worcestershire sauce, and a sprinkle of black pepper. Stir and heat. Add water if needed.

TUNA AND PASTA LA KING

Cut 1 onion and ½ red bell pepper and ½ yellow bell pepper in bite sized pieces and cook in a little oil in a skillet on medium heat until soft. Add 10.5 oz. can of cream of mushroom soup plus ¼ cup milk and a 5 or 6 oz. can of tuna. Stir. Add 1 cup frozen peas, 1 cup cooked whole wheat or brown rice or quinoa spaghetti, and 1 tsp. Worcestershire sauce and sprinkle with black pepper. Add more milk to desired consistency. Heat. Cooked quinoa or brown rice can be used instead of spaghetti. If desired, sprinkle shredded Cheddar cheese on top of each serving. A cup of leftover turkey or chicken can be substituted for the tuna; one large onion and one red bell pepper works well; a little more milk is added.

GROUND TURKEY A LA KING

Cut 1 onion and 1 red and 1 yellow bell pepper into bite sized pieces and cook with 1 minced clove of garlic in oil until fork tender and remove to a plate. Cook 1 lb. thawed ground turkey in same skillet. Add a 10.5 oz. can of Cream of chicken or Cream of Mushroom soup and 1 tsp. Worcestershire sauce. Heat. Add onion and peppers and garlic back in. Heat and serve over baked potato or brown rice or quinoa.

GROUND TURKEY AND VEGETABLES STIR-FRY

Cook 1 green and 1 red bell pepper and 1 large onion cut into bite-sized pieces in a little oil in a skillet on medium heat. Add 2 cups of frozen mixed broccoli, cauliflower, and sliced carrots. When heated through remove to another container. Cook 1 lb. thawed ground turkey, leaving it in chunks. Add 1/8 tsp. ginger, 1/8 tsp. black pepper, 1 tsp. dried parsley, 1 tsp. basil and 5 tsp. soy sauce. When hot add back the vegetables, warm, and serve over brown rice.

GROUND MEAT, VEGETABLE, AND QUINOA MEDLEY

Cut in bite-sized pieces, 3½ red and green bell peppers, 2 medium onion, and 1 zucchini and cook until fork tender with 3 cloves of minced garlic in a little oil in a skillet over medium heat. Remove from skillet to another container and cook 1 lb. of thawed ground turkey or other meat. Add 1 can (14.5 oz.) diced tomatoes, and 1 can (26 oz.) Hunt's Classic Garlic and Herb Spaghetti Sauce or other no white sugar added tomato sauce, 1 cup cooked quinoa, 1 tsp. basil, 1 tsp. oregano, 1/8 tsp. black pepper, 1 tsp. Italian seasoning, and 1 Tbsp. maple syrup or honey. When hot add vegetables back in and bring to a boil and serve.

CHEESE CAKE

Soften 1 envelope of Knox gelatin in ¼ cup of pineapple juice from a 20 oz. can of crushed pineapple in pineapple juice. Put 16 oz. (2 cups) of low fat cottage cheese in blender and blend. Add ¾ cup of drained crushed pineapple, the gelatin in pineapple juice, 1 Tbsp. lemon juice, 1 tsp. vanilla extract, and 1 egg and blend. Pour into a pie pan lined by a whole wheat or other whole-grain crust or pan without crust. Bake at 350 degrees F. for about 45 min. Doubling the recipe uses up the whole can of crushed pineapple in pineapple juice.

FRUIT CAKE

Mix 4¼ cups whole wheat or other whole-grain flour with 1 Tbsp. grated lemon peel, 1 Tbsp. cinnamon, 1 Tbsp. allspice, 1½ tsp. cloves, ¼ tsp. cardamom, and 1 Tbsp. nutmeg. Mix 1 cup of the flour mixture with 1 cup chopped figs, 2 cups chopped dried apricots, 2 cups chopped dried peaches, 2 cups chopped pitted dates, 1 cup dark raisins, 1 cup golden raisins, 1 cup currents, 2 cups chopped walnuts, 2 cups chopped pecans, 2 cups sliced almonds, and 1 cup chopped fresh orange peel from navel oranges. Cream 2 cups butter (1 pound) with 2 Tbsp. Black Strap Molasses, 2 Tbs. vanilla, and 12 egg yolks. Mix in 2 cups drained pineapple tidbits canned in pineapple juice). Alternately add flour mixture and 2 cups fruit juice (pineapple juice from canned pineapple tidbits plus apple or grape juice to make 2 cups). Mix in floured fruit and nut mixture. Beat 12 egg whites until stiff not dry, and fold into batter. A dishpan works well.

Bake in oiled no-stick bakeware (e.g. Bundt or loaf pans) at 275 degrees F. for 1½ hour or until a toothpick comes out clean. Let stand for 30 min. before removing cakes from pans. Wrap in cheesecloth wet with ¼ cup vinegar and ¾ cup apple juice to prevent molding, and plastic bags or Saran wrap and store in refrigerator or freezer.

This makes two 12 cup Bundt cakes + 1 lb. load cake or 6 of the 6 cup Bundt cakes, filled with 3½ cups of batter. Line regular pans with greased and floured paper.

OATMEAL RAISIN AND NUT COOKIES

Mash 3 ripe bananas in a mixing bowl with a fork or potato masher. Add 1/3 cup canola oil, ½ tsp. vanilla, and 1 egg and mix.

Combine 2 cups rolled oats, ¼ cup whole wheat or other whole-grain flour, 1½ tsp. cinnamon, ½ tsp. ginger; then add 1 cup raisins, and 1 cup chopped pecans or walnuts, mix and add to the banana mixture. Mix. Drop by teaspoonful onto greased cookie sheets. Baked at 350 degrees for 22 min. Loosen cookies and let cool on cookie sheets. This makes about 45 cookies.

DARK CHOCOLATE GRANOLA BARS

Combine ¼ cup maple syrup, ¼ cup honey, 2 Tbsp. (1/8 cup) peanut butter, 1 egg, 1 Tbsp. milk, and 1 tsp. vanilla. Combine 1 cup whole wheat or other whole-grain flour, ½ tsp baking soda, 1 tsp cinnamon and ¼ tsp. allspice and add to first mixture. Combine 2 cups old fashioned oats, 1½ cups crisp brown rice cereal, ½ cup dark chocolate chips (1 chipped Bakers unsweetened baking chocolate squares). ¼ cup dried unsweetened cranberries, and ½ cup chopped walnuts and add to above. Mix. I used a flat wooden paddle. Press into a greased 13 x 9 inch baking pan. Bake 18 to 20 min. at 350 degrees F. Cut into 24 bars.

BROWNIES

Beat 4 eggs at room temperature with ¼ tsp. salt. Gradually add 1¼ cup maple syrup and 1 tsp. vanilla and beat until creamy. Heat ¾ cup butter and cool it; stir it and add it to the above mixture. Then fold in a mixture of 1 cup of whole wheat or other whole-grain flour and ¾ cup (12 Tbsp.) cocoa. Stir in gently 1 cup chopped pecans. Bake in a 9 x 13 in. greased baking pan at 350 degrees F for 27 min. or until toothpick comes out clean. Cut into 24 squares.

To substitute honey for maple syrup, use 1 tsp. less than 1¼ cups, and grease or oil the measuring cup so the honey will slip off easily.

PREVENT, REVERSE DIABETES

(GOOD NUTRITION IN A NUTSHELL)

High fiber foods, not processed, is the ounce that prevents. Foods stripped of the way they come from the gardens and the farms are also stripped of their vitamin and mineral content. Only empty calories remain. Without the fiber to slow the absorption high levels of sugar in the blood trigger high levels of insulin which quickly stores the calories for future use in fat. This results in the high rate of too much fat stored in the bodies of children and adults who eat what they find in ample supply in groceries and restaurants. Thus we have high levels of diabetes, heart attacks, strokes and cancer as well as gall stones, hiatus hernia, colon polyps and cancers, sleep apnea, and appendicitis. Indigenous people who eat as their ancestors did have none of these problems, also no arthritis.

Where do we get this life-saving and misery-saving fiber? Products are sold at stores. Better yet eat it. All fruits and vegetables have plenty of fiber naturally. If we buy the juices or squeeze our oranges into juice, we miss the fiber. Also the juices are absorbed rapidly and cause a rapid rise of higher levels of blood sugar than the apple, the orange, the grapes, etc. I've suggested to diabetics to carry tiny boxes of raisins with them instead of candy to eat in case they experience low blood sugar levels. All whole grains are great sources of good fiber. Oatmeal, Brown Rice and 100% Whole Wheat are readily available. Many restaurants offer whole wheat spaghetti or linguini to substitute for the white spaghetti. Beans, peas, lentils, sweet potatoes, peanuts and all vegetables we pull out of the ground such as carrots, onions, rutabagas, turnips, and beets are wonderful, delicious foods full of fiber. Melons such as watermelon, cantaloupe, and honey dew melons and all berries such as gooseberry, currents, raspberries, strawberries, and blueberries are delicious ways to get fiber; also they are very low in calories for those watching their weight. Just think of all the great antioxidants they bring to the table to help our brains and hearts.

So how do we attain a normal weight essential for avoiding diabetes, heart attacks, strokes, many of the cancers, arthritis of the knees, hips, backs and many other ills? We stick to health-giving foods and avoid all items containing white sugar, white flour (enriched means a dollar is removed and a few cents put back), white rice, white flour items such as white pastas (macaroni, spaghetti, shells, tiny pastas added to soups, lasagna, etc.), cookies, cakes, most candies, most pies, tempting desserts. All these items can be made using life-giving ingredients used by our ancestors. In addition to avoiding the calories empty of vitamins, minerals, and fiber, it is important to get protein foods. Protein foods stick to our ribs as my mama would say; they keep the blood sugar at a low even keel and avoid highs and lows. Eggs, cottage cheese, lean meats, fish, poultry such as chicken and turkey, and cheeses are easily available protein foods. Combining nuts or beans or legumes with whole grains provides proteins because they complement each other and together provide all the essential amino acids that make up a complete protein food. Examples are a peanut butter or almond butter sandwich on 100% whole wheat bread, succotash made of whole kernels of corn and lima beans, brown rice and beans, whole grain corn tortillas with beans, pea soup made with brown rice or barley, lentils and brown rice, and soup beans with corn bread. Getting fiber and protein in our tummies 3 or more times a day keeps us from getting hungry and feeling starved, thus avoiding snatching what happens to be handy but may not be health-giving. Fiber keeps us feeling comfortably full.

BIBLIOGRAPHY

Anderson, James W., MD: Diabetes a Practical New Guide to Healthy Living. New York. Warner Brooks, Inc., 1983

Anderson, James W., MD: High Fiber Diet. Department of Medical and Clinical Nutrition, University of Kentucky, Lexington, KY.

Anderson, James W., MD and Breecher, Maury M., MPH, PhD: Live Longer Better. New York. Carroll & Graf Publishers, Inc. 1996

Boonstra, Shawn with Hardinge, Fred, Dr.PH, RD: Easy Steps for Better Health. Nampa, Idaho/Oshawa, Ontario, Pacific Press Publishing Association. 2007.

Burkitt, Denis, MD: Don't Forget Fiber in Your Diet. New York. Arco Publishing, Inc. 1984.

Colbert, Donald, MD: Weight Loss and Muscle Gain. Lake Mary, Florida. Siloam Press

Conn's Current Therapy 2003, edited by Robert E. Rakel, MD and Edward T. Bope, MD. Philadelphia, PA. Saunders Elsevier. 2003.

Conn's Current Therapy 2007, edited by Robert E. Rakel, MD and Edward T. Bope, MD. Philadelphia, PA. Saunders Elsevier. 2007.

Crook, William G., MD: The Yeast Connection. Jackson, Tennessee, Professional Books. 1984.

Davis, Adele, AB, MS: Let's Eat Right to Keep Fit. New York, Harcourt, Brace, and Company. 1954.

Davis Adele, AB, MS: Let's Have Healthy Children. New York Harcourt, Brace, and Company. 1951

Diel, Has, Dr. HS., MPH: Honoring a Scientific Great. Coronary Health Improvement Project (CHIP) regarding the Bower Award awarded to Denis P. Burkitt, MD.

Encyclopaedia Britannica, 1963: Article on Beriberi. England. Encyclopaedia Britannica, Inc., vol 3, pp 506-507.

Harrison's principles of Internal Medicine, 14th edition. New York. McGraw-Hill. 1998.

Haymie, Robert, MD, PhD: A Touch of Soul Cookbook. Cleveland, OH 94106.

Katz, David L., MD, MPH: Nutrition in Clinical Practice. Philadelphia, PA. Lippincott, Williams & Wilkins. 2001.

Ketchum, Katherine and Mueller, L. Ann, MD: Eating Right to Live Sober. Seattle, Madrona Publishers. 1983.

Kirschmann, John D., Director, Nutrition Search, Inc.: Nutrition Almanac. New York. McGraw-Hill Book Company. 1975.

Latham, Michael C., MD et al: Scope Manuel on Nutrition. The Upjohn Company. 1972

Reuben, David, MD: The Save Your Life Diet. La Presa Enterprises, Inc., Random House, Inc., New York and Random House of Canada, LTD., Toronto. 1975.

Rubin, Jordan S.: The Maker's Diet. Lake Mary, FL. Siloam, a Strang Company. 2005.

Salaman, Maureen Kennedy: All Your Health Questions Answered Naturally. MKS, Inc. 1998.

Ser Vaas, Cory, MD: Dr. Denis Burkitt: A Passion for Preventing Disease. Saturday Evening Post. April 1984, pp 67, 96.

Shils, Maurice E., MD, ScD, Olson, James A., PhD, and Shike, Moshe, MD, ed: Modern Nutrition in Health and Disease, eighth edition, vol. 1 & 2. Philadelphia, PA. Lea & Febiger, Williams & Wilkins. 1994.

Voel, Donald and Judith: Biochemistry, Second Edition. New York. John Wiley and Sons, Inc. 1995.

Yeager, Selene and the editors of Prevention Health Books: The Doctor's Book of Food Remedies. Rodale, Inc. 1998.

www.ingramcontent.com/pod-product-compliance
Ingram Content Group UK Ltd.
Pitfield, Milton Keynes, MK11 3LW, UK
UKHW041954230426
12048UKWH00008B/335